Development and Disorders of Speech in Childhood

Publication Number 614
AMERICAN LECTURE SERIES®

A Monograph in
The BANNERSTONE DIVISION *of*
AMERICAN LECTURES IN SPEECH AND HEARING

Edited by
ROBERT W. WEST
Visiting Professor of Speech
University of California
Los Angeles, California

Development and Disorders of Speech in Childhood

Fourth Printing

By

ISAAC W. KARLIN, B.S., M.D., F.A.A.P.

Late Attending Pediatrician and Physician-in-charge, Speech Clinic, Jewish Hospital of Brooklyn (New York); Consulting Pediatrician, National Hospital for Speech Disorders, New York, New York; Consultant in Speech Rehabilitation, Jewish Chronic Disease Hospital, Brooklyn, New York

DAVID B. KARLIN, A.B., M.D., M.Sc. (Ophth.)

Assistant Attending Ophthalmic Surgeon, The Mount Sinai Hospital; Associate Attending Ophthalmic Surgeon, Manhattan Eye, Ear and Throat Hospital, New York, New York; Ophthalmic Medical Adviser to the New York City Director, Selective Service System

LOUISE GURREN, A.B., M.A., Ph.D.

Professor of Speech Education, New York University, New York, New York; Former Director of the Bureau for Speech Improvement, Board of Education, City of New York

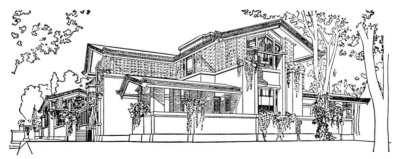

CHARLES C THOMAS • PUBLISHER

Springfield • Illinois • U.S.A.

Published and Distributed Throughout the World by

CHARLES C THOMAS • PUBLISHER

BANNERSTONE HOUSE

301-327 East Lawrence Avenue, Springfield, Illinois, U.S.A.

© *1965 by* CHARLES C THOMAS • PUBLISHER

ISBN 0-398-00973-2

Library of Congress Catalog Card Number: 65-11688

First Printing, 1965
Second Printing, 1970
Third Printing, 1973
Fourth Printing, 1977

With THOMAS BOOKS careful attention is given to all details of manufacturing and design. It is the Publisher's desire to present books that are satisfactory as to their physical qualities and artistic possibilities and appropriate for their particular use. THOMAS BOOKS will be true to those laws of quality that assure a good name and good will.

Printed in the United States of America
00-2

DEDICATION

Isaac W. Karlin, B.S., M.D., F.A.A.P.

(1897-1962)

This book is dedicated to the memory of Isaac W. Karlin, pediatrician and pioneer in the diagnosis and treatment of speech disorders in children.

Karlin made a unique contribution to the field of language problems in children by combining his knowledge of medicine with speech pathology. As a practicing pediatrician, Karlin was interested in not only the physical health of the child, but in his emotional, intellectual, and language development as well. He was one of the first founders and organizers of a speech clinic in a hospital setting in this country. In 1916, the first classes for the speech handicapped were organized in the public schools of the City of New York. During the first part of the twentieth century, speech therapy was mainly the province of speech specialists and educators. In recognition of the close association of language development with the physical growth and development of the child, Karlin founded, organized, and directed the first hospital-affiliated speech clinic at the Jewish Hospital of Brooklyn in 1940.

Karlin first introduced his *Psychosomatic Theory of Stuttering* in the *Journal of Speech Disorders* in 1947. In the course of his work, he obtained several grants from the National Institutes of Health and the Office of Vocational Rehabilitation to study language disability in the aphasic and in the mentally retarded.

After Karlin received his degree of Doctor of Medicine from Illinois in 1924, he did postgraduate work in neuropsychiatry at the College of Physicians and Surgeons, Columbia University. Karlin practiced pediatrics in Brooklyn, New York, from 1925 to the close of his life. He was an assistant instructor in neurology at the College of Physicians and Surgeons, Columbia University, from 1931 to 1935; taught undergraduate and graduate speech courses at Brooklyn College in 1954; and was Assistant Clinical Professor at Yale University School of Medicine during 1956-1958. In 1960, he was a lecturer and participant at the Institute of Childhood Aphasia of Stanford University School of Medicine.

In 1960, Karlin arranged with Gurren, for the publication of a book on speech and language disorders in children, that would be a compilation of his work as well as that of other authorities in the field. Due to his death in 1962, Karlin wrote only a few chapters. The present authors have completed the book, using his publications, lectures, and notes as well as contributing from their own experience and knowledge in the field. Furthermore, in order to present current ideas on the subject, the authors have included the work of other investigators in the field of speech pathology.

It is the hope of the authors that this book will serve as an appropriate tribute to the life and work of Isaac W. Karlin.

DAVID B. KARLIN, M.D.
LOUISE GURREN, PH.D.

PREFACE

THIS BOOK discusses the growth, development, and abnormalities of speech in childhood from the pediatric point of view. It is partly an outgrowth of articles, lectures, and experiences of the authors during years of work with children having speech problems. The text is written from both the medical and educational approaches. In addition, the authors have included much of the recent thinking on the part of other authorities in the field of speech pathology.

This book embodies four main purposes in dealing with language in childhood. The first aspect describes the normal course and development of speech and language from its origin in infancy through its maturation during adolescence. A second purpose is to present the anatomical, physiological, and psychological aspects of the speech mechanism. The third aim is to explain, according to present knowledge in the field, the causes of both organic and functional (including emotional) speech and language disorders. Fourthly, suggestions for speech therapy are given for each type of disturbance. The educational, as well as the medical and clinical approaches to helping children with speech and language problems, are also discussed.

The material is presented in a form that can be understood not only by the medical and educational professionals in the field, but equally as well by parents and others who are not working directly in the area of speech. Normal anatomical and physiological development is presented first, because only after one becomes conversant with the normal mechanism of speech can one view the pathology of speech production.

Medical investigators recognize the fact that problems arising during adult life frequently can be traced to difficulties encountered during childhood development. This is certainly true for psychiatric disturbances. Similarly, many of the speech and language difficulties of the adult have their inception during childhood. The underlying goal of this book is to provide an awareness of causes and treatment of childhood speech defects, in an attempt to prevent more serious communicative problems in one's more productive adult life.

It is hoped that the readers of this book will be stimulated toward further investigative research and the expansion of both clinical and educational speech therapy facilities for the child. Furthermore, it is the authors' desire that through this book, medical students, pediatricians, speech clinicians, educators, and parents will gain a deeper understanding of the speech development and problems in childhood.

The authors gratefully acknowledge the constructive suggestions offered by Dr. Robert West, Editor of the American Lecture Series in Speech and Hearing, and Professor of Speech, University of California at Los Angeles. The writers are also appreciative of the helpful suggestions made in the field of audiology by Dr. Maurice Miller, Assistant Professor of Clinical Otolaryngology, New York University School of Medicine. The authors also wish to express their appreciation to the many publishers who have so generously given permission for the use of illustrations. They are indebted to the many investigators in the field of speech and language whose works have been quoted herein.

A grateful acknowledgment is given to Mr. Robert Carlin who so skillfully prepared the photographs of the illustrations, and to Miss Irene Musil who was responsible for the typing of the manuscript. Dr. David Karlin also wishes to thank his wife, Adrienne, for her understanding and encouragement during the writing of this book.

DAVID B. KARLIN, M.D.
LOUISE GURREN, PH.D.

CONTENTS

Development and Disorders of Speech in Childhood

Part I

ORIGIN AND NORMAL DEVELOPMENT OF
SPEECH AND LANGUAGE

Chapter 1

THEORIES OF THE ORIGIN OF SPEECH AND LANGUAGE IN MAN

Speech is characteristically and distinctly a human function. Apart from the mechanical noises made by many animals, no form of life lower than the amphibians is capable of making laryngeal sounds. With birds, however, there is a great advance in sounds which foreshadow the production of vowels. Even the parrot, who supposedly produces intelligent speech, is capable of making only certain noises. These noises appear to the human brain as reproductions of sounds made by man in the production of speech. The mammals show no advance over lower animals in the production of sound. Yet, because of their larger brain, the mammals possess two important elements of language: the involuntary cry of emotion and the voluntary cry of warning. Thus, mammals convey limited messages, although their cries do not possess the faculty of symbolization characteristic of human language.

Recent observations by von Frisch (1) disclose an elaborate system of gestural communication in the social insects. In the bee, at least, communication as concise and explicit as a system of naval signals dominates social organization. Although Revesz (2) denies the relevance of "animal language" to the understanding of human speech, animal communication is accepted today as a biological fact of first importance by Zangwill (3). Peterson (4), a noted ornithologist, states that there is truly such a thing as "the language of the birds." Some of it is innate and some of it is acquired. Can one ever understand this "language"?

Speech, unlike almost all other human activities, has left no record of its origin and development. The mystery of the origin of speech is veiled in the origin of the human race. Many theories of the origin of speech and language have been formulated. Yet, none has proved adequate in providing a satisfactory explanation.

5

Hieroglyphics, the earliest drawings and writings, are valuable in explaining man's history. They indicate, however, that complex symbolic processes had already been developed and that the beginnings of speech had long been passed. The fact that the origin of speech goes far back beyond recorded human history, indicates that any attempt at explanation must be theoretical.

THEORIES OF ORIGIN OF SPEECH

The theories of the origin of speech and language can be divided into the earlier hypotheses and the later theories with their attempted, more scientific, explanations. To the earlier group of theories belong the divine origin theory, the onomatopoetic theory and the interjectional theory. Later day work was responsible for the gesture theory with its modifications, as well as the most advanced psychological and philological explanations.

Divine Origin Theory

The earliest theory of speech is that of *divine origin.* The theory is expounded by theologians and philosophers. It is stated in Genesis (5), "And whatsoever Adam called every living creature, that was the name thereof." It is of interest to note that the Bible also speaks of the origin of the various languages throughout the world. In the beginning, the whole earth was of one language and of one speech. As the sons of Noah journeyed east, they decided to build a city with a tower reaching toward heaven. The Lord then decided to, "confound their language that they may not understand one another's speech." The tower was called Babel and the Lord, "scattered the people abroad upon the face of the earth."

One notes in literature that belief in divine origin of speech is not limited to Judeo-Christian theology. Other races and other tribes had their own legends touching upon the beginnings of language. To the Norsemen, speech was a gift handed down by Thor, the God of Thunder.

Onomatopoetic Theory

Lefèvre's (6) *onomatopoetic theory* assumes that primitive words arose in imitation of various natural sounds, such as the barking of dogs and the crackling of fire. Although onomatopoetic words comprise only a small portion of human speech, they do form a significant group in the vocabulary of the small child. Lefèvre (6) traces the origin of speech back to the human cry and still further back to the animal cry. Although it has been shown that some primitive tribes speak languages in which onomatopoetic words are totally absent, this theory does account for a part of the origin of articulate communication.

Interjectional Theory

The *interjectional theory* of Judd (7) is based upon the belief that the earliest speech sounds were involuntary exclamations brought about through emotional excitement such as joy, fear, sorrow, and astonishment. The usual interjections are abrupt expressions for sudden sensations and emotions. They represent a reflex process with a highly emotional overtone. Thus, an interjection may serve the purpose of communication or warning, as when the instinctive cry of a frightened animal puts the herd to flight. The interjectional theory attributes the derivation of language to the emotions common to both man and animal.

The onomatopoetic and interjectional theories fail to consider speech as a form of social intercourse, as a means of communication between man and his neighbor. To explain the purpose of speech and language as a means of communication, one must consider the psychological gesture theory of Wundt (8), the oral gesture theory of Paget (9), the philological vocal play theory of Jespersen (10), and the social control theory of de Laguna (11).

Gesture Theory

The *gesture theory* of Wundt (8) of the origin of speech is based on the psychological law that every sensation has its own distinct expression. Each sensation is brought about through nerve connections between organs that receive a stimulus (receptors) and those that respond to the stimulus (effectors). In other words, a stimulus or a gesture, such as touching the finger to the eye, causes blinking. Not only does the action serve a particular individual in the form of a definite sensation, but it causes similar feelings to be present in other persons. Physical contact, as shown in the above example, is not necessary as a means of communication. Gesture language can aid in the communication of ideas by different movements of the hands and arms as well as by the accompaniment of facial expressions. The gesture theory emphasizes that speech is basically a communicative function.

Gestural communication is useful to man today in spite of the higher development of oral language. In the process of evolution, the articulate language displaced the more primitive gesture language because of its greater flexibility. This evolutionary process freed both arms and eyes for functions required in man's struggle for existence. It is also possible that gesture and the spoken word came to be used simultaneously in the very earliest period of speech, supporting and supplementing each other. Finally, sound language gained the upper hand and gradually put gestures into the background without completely eliminating them. The gesture theory would indicate that human society was already highly organized when speech began and that gestures evolved from the existence of ideas which individuals desired to communicate.

Oral Gesture Theory

The *oral gesture theory* of Paget (9) proceeds from the gesture period to the consideration that when man invented tools, his hands, being occupied with construction, could no longer be used for the communication of ideas. Gestures were now transferred to movements of the mouth, tongue, and lips. Man accompanied the oral gestures with vocalization so that the gestures became audible.

Why has man universally used sound-speech addressing itself to the ear, rather than pictorial or gesture-speech addressing itself to the eye? Darwin (12) reasons that since the hands were employed in gestural speech, they could not be used for other necessary work. Vocal speech, however, frees the hands for other useful functions. Oral speech is also a more universal medium of communication than gesture speech, since sound radiates from the speaker in all directions.

Vocal Play Theory

To coordinate the gesture theories with the earlier, more primitive onomatopoetic and interjectional sound theories, the *vocal play theory* of Jespersen (10) was developed. This theory postulates that the source of speech is the sounds and motions of happy, primitive youths, out of which grew primitive language. Similarly, according to Darwin (12), the origin of language is to be found in the musical exclamations of men before they learned to talk. Darwin (12) believes that bird sounds constitute, in many respects, the closest analogy to language.

This doctrine of priority of song is amplified by Jespersen (10) who believes that primitive speech originates from powerful emotions such as love. Love, in turn, elicits outbursts of music and song. The vocal play theory contends that primitive speech resembles the prelinguistic period of the baby with its humming and cooing. Jespersen (10) feels that speech has largely developed from the association of powerful emotions (one of which is love) which give rise to articulate communication. It is also true that present day languages each exhibit a melody of their own.

Social Control Theory

The *social control theory* of de Laguna (11) regards the development of speech as an instrument of human cooperation in a society that gradually became more complex and required concerted cooperation for survival. "Speech is the great medium through which human cooperation is brought about. It is the means by which the activities of man are coordinated with each other for the attainment of common aims."

According to de Laguna (11), the increasing complexity of life and the need for protection, make necessary cooperative measures for existence. Hunting, agriculture, the use of tools, all make desirable a new instrument of social expression designed for both protection and cooperation. Thus, the change in social conditions toward the more complex forms is accompanied by the need for more effective means of social control. Therefore, speech follows the evolutionary progress of man.

COMPARISON OF LANGUAGE DEVELOPMENT IN CHILDREN WITH THE ORIGIN OF LANGUAGE

Attempts have been made to compare the earliest stages of linguistic development in the human race with the development of speech in the child.

Speech development in the child depends upon mental growth. This factor is also operable in the linguistic development of mankind. However, in children the linguistic function is expressed first in the understanding of language or words. The child derives his speech from pre-existing and mature forms of surrounding adult language. This means that the child's speech cannot represent the archaic form of speech that mankind once demonstrated.

COMPARISON OF APHASIC PHENOMENA WITH THE ORIGIN OF LANGUAGE IN MANKIND AND THE DEVELOPMENT OF LANGUAGE IN THE CHILD

Another attempt has been made to reconstruct the development of language from a study of the relearning process in the aphasic individual. It has been said that in the re-acquisition of speech by the aphasic, the aphasic person goes through the evolution and development of speech exhibited by mankind. In other words, as man learned to symbolize and to associate sounds with certain concepts, so the aphasic has to relearn to symbolize.

The assumption is also made that the relearning of language in the aphasic proceeds through similar steps as organization of language in children. Some investigators assume that the possible restitution of speech in aphasics, to some extent, recapitulates the main stages in the development of the child's speech. The aphasic uses the asyntactic speech of one-word sentences. He strings together single words without grammatical construction or syntactical order. He often demonstrates sound reversals and substitutions common in the child. There is also some similarity between the initial learning of speech in the child and the initial relearning process in the aphasic.

One must bear in mind, however, that aphasic phenomena are a result of cortical pathology, a pathology producing *disintegration* of function. The brain damage reduces the aphasic's capacity to make necessary adjustments. Contrary to this, in the child, one is dealing with a process of normal growth and development, implying increasing *integration*. The differences between the personalities of children and those of the aphasic adults may also produce essential differences.

SPEECH AND LANGUAGE

The terms speech and language are frequently used interchangeably. To be exact, however, one must differentiate between speech and language.

Speech, in the sense that its purpose is to convey ideas and thoughts, is a form of language communication. However, the distinct feature of speech is the faculty of uttering articulate *sounds*. The emission of sounds produced in the larynx and modified by the accessory structures of the throat, mouth, and nasal cavities finally give rise to what one considers to be speech. Speech is a verbal process, a means of oral communication between one individual and another.

Language is a psychic process, centered in the brain. In its widest sense, language signifies the expression of thoughts and ideas. The sign language used by the American Indian, the manual communication of the deaf mute, or the language of the eyes, is language just as much as verbal communication. Although sign language can convey varied thought processes, its most severe limitation is that the speaker and the person receiving the communication must be in visual contact with each other.

Primitive language is mediated by postures, by facial expressions, gestures, and sound formations. In animals as well as in man, postures indicate feelings or moods, such as the extended limbs, arched back, erect fur and lashing tail of an outraged cat.

Gestures such as the pricking up of the ears and movements of the head in the act of listening, are further examples. The production of sounds exhibited by early man is that form of language leading toward speech.

It is evident that the origin of speech lies so far back in human history that it is impossible to achieve factual certainty. None of the previously stated theories can totally explain the beginnings of speech and language as one knows it today. Yet, each adds to the appearance of certain elements of human speech. Words, as part of human thought, may be regarded as living, protean entities. They grow, take root, and adapt themselves to environmental changes like plants and animals. Speech has as its purpose, the establishment of mental contact among men. It develops gradually with the expansion of the human brain and the increasingly complex social life. One thing is certain, however. Speech has developed as a process of evolution rather than as a chance occurrence.

REFERENCES

(1) von Frisch, K.: *The Dancing Bees.* London, Methuen & Co., 1954.

(2) Revesz, G.: *Origins and Prehistory of Language.* Translated from the German by Butler, J., London, Longmans, 1956.

(3) Zangwill, O. L.: Speech. In Field, J. ed.: *Handbook of Physiology, Neurophysiology, Vol. 3.* Washington, D. C., American Physiological Society, 1960.

(4) Peterson, R. T.: Why Birds Sing, and What. *New York Times Magazine, October 22,* 1961.

(5) *The Bible, King James Version.* Philadelphia, Jewish Publication Society of America, 1944.

(6) Lefèvre, A.: *Race and Language.* New York, Appleton-Century Co., 1894.

(7) Judd, C. H.: *The Psychology of Social Institutions.* New York, The Macmillan Co., 1926.

(8) Wundt, W.: *Elements of Folk Psychology.* Translated by Schaub, E. L., London, G. Allen & Unwin Ltd., 1916.

(9) Paget, R.: *Human Speech.* New York, Harcourt, Brace & Co., 1930.

(10) Jespersen, O.: *Language; Its Nature, Development and Origin.* New York, Henry Holt, 1922.

(11) de Laguna, G. A.: *Speech; Its Function and Development.* New Haven, Yale University Press, 1927.

(12) Darwin, C.: *The Descent of Man and Selection in Relation to Sex.* London, J. Murray, 1871.

Chapter 2

DEVELOPMENT OF SPEECH
AND LANGUAGE IN THE CHILD

IT IS WELL to understand the nature of speech and language and the development in the human race in order to trace the growth of the child's ability to communicate through speech.

The various theories of the origin of language have been discussed. Investigators agree that even the most primitive tribe has a systematic series of spoken symbols that convey meaning to the listener. Sapir (1) states that, "Of all aspects of culture, it is a fair guess that language was the first to receive a highly developed form and that its essential perfection is a prerequisite to the development of culture as a whole."

NATURE OF SPEECH AND LANGUAGE

Speech may be described as a structural system of arbitrary vocal sounds and sequences of sounds which are used in communication. The sounds, put together in certain order, symbolize meanings. Spoken language has both *acoustic* and *word structures* which must be mastered for ordinary communication.

First, the *acoustic or phonetic* structure is composed of the following: articulation of the sounds of the language, duration or length of sound, syllable division, stress on syllables of words, stress on words in groups, phrasing or grouping of words according to meaning, and intonation. Each of these elements plays an important semantic role in the speaker's communication. Each language has its own system of sounds, its way of dividing syllables, and its stress on syllables of words, both as to location and degree. In regard to stress on words in groups, most languages select for stress the key words in a group, but some languages have much lighter stress than others. Languages vary in length of phrase or thought groups. Every language has a distinct intonation of its own.

14

The second element of spoken language involves word structure. It concerns *syntax* or the placing of words in a certain order, *morphology* or using appropriate endings to qualify the meaning of words, and *vocabulary* or the choice of words to convey the desired meaning. This choice of words implies a reservoir of "inner language" which may be drawn upon as the speaker desires. The speaker composes phrases and utters them without selecting each individual word and putting it in the proper structural pattern.

How does the child use the phonetic and word pattern structures to communicate with those around him? How does he learn the meanings of words? How does he connect the sounds he hears and voices with the meanings?

The growth of the child's ability to speak is of utmost importance to his future functioning as a thinking, educable human being. Language is the instrument of thought, communication, and learning. How the child acquires speech divides itself into two aspects: the *comprehension* and the *production* of language.

FIRST SOUNDS

For purposes of speech development, the term infancy refers to the period in the child's life before he begins to talk. The word infancy is derived from the Latin *in* (without) and *fari* (to speak). The first sound the infant utters is the birth cry. Cases are reported, however, of fetal crying known as *vagitus uterinus.* This sound is the premature cry of the fetus before the head appears. It may take place under the following circumstances: rupture of the fetal membranes; entrance of air into the birth canal making it available to fetal inspiration; stimulation of the fetal respiratory center. Theoretically, intrauterine crying suggests danger of the fetus drowning in amniotic fluid. This is not the case, however, since the membranes are ruptured and the fluid drained away. Vagitus uterinus should be considered a danger signal because it may precede the beginning of fetal asphyxia. One half to three hours may elapse between the infant's crying *in utero* and his delivery in good condition.

The birth cry is the first and most primitive process of phonation. This sound is the result of a reflex, involuntary action. It has a crucial physiological function. Since crying consists of deep inspiration followed by a prolonged expiration, causing vibrations of the vocal cords, the first cry establishes normal respiration for the oxygenation of blood.

The first cries may also have diagnostic values. One may distinguish the healthy, vigorous cry of the full-term newborn from the weak, whining cry of the premature infant. Another type of cry, a stridulous sound, may indicate laryngeal obstruction. There is also the hoarse, harsh cry of the cretin. The cephalic cry (high-pitched, plaintive, and piercing) takes place during sleep and then ceases as suddenly as it begins. This type of cry may indicate increased intracranial pressure.

Newborn babies spend about two hours a day crying. The amount of crying is in inverse ratio to the amount of nursing care that the baby receives. While it might be desirable to reduce crying time to a minimum, a certain amount is necessary to stimulate vocal and respiratory functions. Within the first few weeks, cries begin to be differentiated by shades of loudness and even by tone. The hungry baby screams. The same infant, with colic when he cries, makes sounds with a different quality. Infants soon learn that crying or screaming brings response from their surroundings, thus making it possible to control the environment.

During the first year, in addition to expressing pain or discomfit, the infant gradually learns how to convey pleasure through smiling. Toward the end of the year, he begins to laugh, thereby expressing an entirely new type of sound.

BABBLING—PLAYING WITH SOUNDS

In the development of speech, the child moves through the following stages of communication: screaming time; crowing and babbling time; talking time. During the pre-linguistic period the infant uses what Jespersen (2) calls his own "little language." Later the child uses the "common language," the language of the community.

While crying exercises only the vocal cords and the breathing mechanism, babbling exercises not only the voice and respiratory mechanisms, but the lips and tongue as well. Early babbling is

a *reflex* phenomenon while late babbling is a *circular* phenomenon. Babbling becomes a circular phenomenon not only because
of the child's enjoyment of the kinesthetic pleasure of exercising
his lips and tongue, but also as a result of the pleasure of hearing
the sounds he himself produces. It is as though he enjoys hearing
himself say a certain sound so much that he repeats it over and
over just for the joy of hearing himself say it. The deaf child
will also begin to babble in the early, reflex manner. Because
he lacks the feedback stimulus of hearing himself produce sounds,
he babbles less and less, and finally ceases to do so. The hard-
of-hearing, lacking an adequate feedback mechanism, does not
obtain the pleasure from babbling which is so essential for the
further development of speech.

Seth and Guthrie (3) state that during the first few months of
life, although the infant hears sounds, he is not capable of sound
discrimination. Later, as soon as he begins to discriminate sound
and can see the movements of the speaker's lips and tongue, he
tries to imitate what he sees and hears. It is difficult to state
accurately the importance of the visual aspect in speech development. One knows that comprehension is greatly aided by seeing
the speaker. The child imitates gestures he sees. It is therefore
safe to assume that the infant, seeing movements of the lips and
jaws of speakers around him, is stimulated to imitate them. Thus,
the infant is stimulated by the auditory, kinesthetic, and visual
aspects of speech.

Inarticulate babbling or playing with sounds, continues for
some time. During this play period, the infant does not necessarily produce sounds of his own language. An infant, observed
by Gurren, practiced a nasal, palatalized consonant followed by
a vowel for an entire morning. This particular consonant is
used in Russian (in Lenin). The baby who enjoyed hearing
himself say the sound, however, lived in an all-English speaking
home and community.

During this period of the child's growth it is important for
him to hear sounds from adults and children around him. Thus,
the babbling of the infant will begin to sound more and more
like the speech he hears. Even before the infant begins to use

the sounds of his language, he will begin to imitate the intonation around him. Thus, his babbling gradually assumes a tone different from his earlier, reflex phonation.

FIRST SPEECH SOUNDS

In the acquisition of speech, it would appear that the infant's perception of his own speech sounds plays a most important part in governing motor development. Indeed, "circular reactions" are readily set up in which a speech sound, once spoken, initiates its own repetition. This process no doubt provides the basis for imitation and repetition of the speech of others. The ear-voice "feedback loop," it appears, is of the utmost importance in the monitoring of speech and in providing the basis for orderly speech development.

The first aspect of the phonetic structure of language mentioned earlier in this chapter is the articulation of the sounds of speech, i.e., consonants and vowels, including diphthongs (two vowels blended into one). Apparently, since vowels have a higher acoustic perceptibility than consonants, these sounds are uttered first. The child's first consonants are usually labials, sounds made with the lips. There are three possible reasons for this. First, the child can see lip consonants made by those in his environment. Second, the infant's lips have had considerable muscular development through sucking. Third, the lip sounds are relatively simple neurologically, being innervated chiefly by one pair of nerves, the seventh cranial. Cerebral palsied children, for example, who have poor muscular coordination of the lips and who cannot pronounce the labial consonants, are given sucking exercises to strengthen the lip muscles so that they may learn to say the sounds *p*, *b*, and *m* more clearly.

The production of the other phonetic elements of language such as stress and intonation are purely spontaneous at the outset. The child is still playing with these aspects of sounds as well as with articulation. Stress, for example, means extra force or greater volume on a syllable or syllables in a group of words. Intonation, or the melody of language, is the rise and fall of the voice. The infant enjoys varying the volume and pitch of his voice.

After the period of pure spontaneity, there is a period of selection of sound combined with the use of stress and intonation. It has been noted that some children use stress and intonation to carry their meaning before they use articulate speech. For example, Gurren observed a two and one-half-year-old boy "scold" his sister. James had been given a toy when he visited relatives with his parents. When they were going home the child's sister, aged five, reminded him to take the toy. James had not forgotten his toy. He had every intention of taking it. He told this to his sister using gestures, stress, and intonation, although his speech was inarticulate. There were no recognizable words, but James communicated most effectively. His sister understood exactly what he said and so did the other members of the audience.

As the child's auditory mechanism records more and more accurately what is heard in his environment, he slowly discards those sounds that are not used around him. During the second half of the first year of life, children have a strong impulse to imitate sounds. They repeat again and again the sounds they hear. This is a very different stage from the purely spontaneous early babbling of the vocal play type. The imitative stage may be considered a form of vocal play with the added pleasure of the fun of imitation.

In the discussion of speech thus far, the all-important matter of meaning has not been discussed. How does the child associate meaning with sound?

SOUND AND MEANING

It is important to keep in mind that during the first year of vocal play and imitation, the child is slowly beginning to understand the speech of those around him. He *comprehends* speech before he himself *produces* articulate speech. The first stage in the comprehension of speech is the association of certain sounds with visual, tactile, and other sensations aroused by objects in the external world. These associations are "stored" as memories. Thus, the child acquires an ever-increasing reservoir of words, a vocabulary of "inner language" upon which he will later draw to express his thoughts.

After meanings are attached to certain spoken words, pathways become established between the cortical auditory area and the motor area for the muscles of articulation. The child then attempts to articulate words from the sounds that he has heard. This act of verbal expression involves the coordinated movements of a large group of respiratory, laryngeal, pharyngeal, lingual, and labial muscles. Later, as the child is taught to read, auditory speech is associated with the visual symbols of speech called letters. Finally, the child learns to express himself by means of the written word through a visual association between letters and the motor area for the hand.

Some children respond to their own names early in the second half of the first year. During the period of babbling and vocal play, there is a slow accumulation of words that are understood but not spoken by the child. These words are gathered from speech in the child's surroundings. The child's understanding of words is greatly enhanced by the use of gestures. The child responds to the words, "come to mother," by toddling to her because she always holds out her arms to him as she repeats the words. In many instances small children can grasp the general meaning of relatively long sentences. The comprehension of sentences is aided by the child's understanding of key words and by gestures used by the speaker.

After the child has connected meaning with sound, and has succeeded in understanding not only single words but sentences as well, he begins to use articulate sounds to convey meaning to others. During this period of gradual comprehension of the speech of others, before the child can speak himself, he "invents" words for objects around him. Sometimes he may use a syllable such as "la." This may mean *food* or *light* or a *toy*. Here the child is associating meaning with his own sounds. Often his listeners pick up the "invented" word and use it with the child. According to Jespersen (4), this is most helpful in aiding the child to connect sounds with meaning in order to identify objects or persons around him.

Usually the child says his first recognizable (non-invented) words by ten to eighteen months of age (see Table I). The rate

TABLE I

TIME OF APPEARANCE OF THE FIRST SPOKEN WORD (DATA FROM BATEMAN)

Age (Months)	Number of Children Using First Word		Total
	Boys	Girls	
8	1	0	1
9	1	4	5
10	1	10	11
11	2	4	6
12	1	2	3
13	3	2	5
14	2	1	3
15	1	0	1
Total	12	23	35

From George Seth and Douglas Guthrie's *Speech in Childhood,* 1935. Courtesy of Oxford University Press, London, England.

of accumulation of spoken words, that is, the rate of increase in vocabulary, is dependent upon many factors in the child's natural endowments and in his environment. Factors in the development of vocabulary will be discussed in the next chapter. There is a tremendous acceleration in the child's production of distinguishable words between the ages of two and one-half and three years. Seth and Guthrie (3) summarized the work of Smith, Gerlach, and Nice showing the growth in the child's vocabulary. Table II shows their results.

It is necessary to remember that the child is learning many other skills during the period of speech and language development. The most important of these is walking. The tremendous effort put forth in learning the muscular coordination and the balance necessary for locomotion may, in some children, temporarily affect language and speech development. Thus, a youngster who has difficulty in learning to walk, may experience emotional stress which may briefly retard speech development.

WIDENING HORIZONS IN SPEECH AND LANGUAGE

At the very beginning, oral communication is used by the child to get what he needs. During the second year, the child's

TABLE II

Average Size of Vocabularies of Children up to Six Years of Age

	Smith		Gerlach		Nice	
Age	No. of Cases	Vocab-ulary	No. of Cases	Vocab-ulary	No. of Cases	Vocab-ulary
1.0	52	3				
1.6	14	22	14	12.5		
2.0	25	272				
2.6	14	446	29	263	25	508
3.0	20	896				
3.6	26	1,222	6	1,190.5	11	1,338
4.0	26	1,540				
4.6	32	1,870	2	1,445 (av.)	7	1,843
5.0	20	2,072				
5.6	27	2,289	2	4,118.5 (av.)	2	4,225
6.0	9	2,562				
6.6	....	....	....	....	2	3,103

From George Seth and Douglas Guthrie's *Speech in Childhood,* 1935. Courtesy of Oxford University Press, London, England.

world widens considerably. This period is characterized by questions about objects. "What's that?" the child asks incessantly as he constantly becomes aware of new objects. He now knows that each of these concrete forms has a name, and that that name always has the same sounds. Thus, he increases the words he says. He adds to his daily usable vocabulary. For example, a three-year-old points up to the sky and says, "What's that?" He listens as his mother says, "A helicopter." He runs immediately to inform his older brothers and sisters that the object in the sky is a "helicopter." The child repeats the word many times with great enjoyment. The fact that it is a polysyllabic word does not trouble him since he is used to saying polysyllabic phrases such as, "Me go out now." He has just added another word to his rapidly increasing vocabulary.

Therefore, during the third year, the child not only becomes aware of the meaning of words, but he says them as well. During this period he also begins to use the speech patterns of his community, in sound, structure, and vocabulary.

BUILDING LANGUAGE STRUCTURE

The nature of language has been described earlier. In addition to being able to convey meaning through sound, the child must master the structural patterns of the language. After he has increased his vocabulary simply by finding out names of concrete objects, he must begin to learn the other types of words: verbs, adjectives, adverbs, connectives, and articles. Furthermore, since one does not talk in single words, but rather in phrases and sentences, it is essential for the child to learn to use this type of structure for communication. The child has successfully used one-word sentences in the past. "Me" may mean "Take me too" or "Give it to me." Gradually, he begins to acquire a feeling for the structural pattern of his language as he learns meanings of words and how to say them.

The child, when grouping words to form sentences, must use the word order that is characteristic of his language. For example, a child in a Spanish environment will hear, "the house white" (la casa blanca), while a child living in an English-speaking community will hear, "the white house." This word order is gathered by ear from the speech of those in the child's environment. The child must also acquire the inflected forms that are characteristic of his language. He must use plurals when he means more than one. He must know that certain endings are characteristic of verbs for denoting person, number, and time or tense. All of these aspects of his language are absorbed by the child through hearing the patterns of speech around him.

It is important to remember that even during the inarticulate period the child talks in phrases and sentences in his own jargon. Earlier in this chapter a "scolding" given by James to his sister is described. This communication is composed of unrecognizable words strung together into phrases and sentences. For development into articulate sentence form, one must wait until the child has a vocabulary of about 150 words. The child usually begins to form sentences between the ages of two and one-half and three years, the period of great increase in vocabulary. Table III shows the development of sentence structure from two to five years of age. Even though the child may try to use connected speech with distinguishable words, he may not use the correct word order at first. He may say a sentence like the following, "Away me went car." It is natural that the child learns nouns first since he begins by asking questions about objects. However, he soon learns verbs of action from those around him. "Clap hands," "pick up," "go down," "go bye-bye" are readily acquired.

TABLE III

DEVELOPMENT OF THE SENTENCE FROM 2 TO 5 YEARS (SMITH)

Age Years, Months	Number of Cases	Words per Sentence (Average)
2.0	11	1.7
2.6	18	2.4
3.0	17	3.3
3.6	23	4.0
4.0	17	4.3
4.6	22	4.7
5.0	16	4.6

From George Seth and Douglas Guthrie's *Speech in Childhood*, 1935. Courtesy of Oxford University Press, London, England.

By three years of age the child usually becomes aware of inflectional changes. He composes some of his own, based on other endings he has heard. He may say "worser," "gooder," and "flied" in an attempt to communicate more shades of meaning than he had before. On the other hand, pronouns, prepositions, and connectives do not appear until articulate speech and some of the structural patterns have been acquired.

The speech development of the child is dependent upon many factors which will be considered in later chapters. Usually the normal child utters his first words by ten to eighteen months of age. If a child fails to speak by the age of three years, he is probably handicapped emotionally, intellectually, or physically. It must be kept in mind, however, that children develop speech at varied rates. Some are quite silent for a long time. They may babble, but they omit the word stage and suddenly blossom forth using phrases and sentences. Carroll (5) says, "By the age of six the average child has mastered nearly all of the phonemic distinctions of his language and practically all its common grammatical forms in construction, at least those used by the adult and older children in his environment."

REFERENCES

(1) Sapir, E.:*Language; An Introduction to the Study of Speech.* New York, Harcourt, Brace & Co., 1921.

(2) Jespersen, O.: *Growth and Structure of the English Language.* New York, Doubleday Anchor Books, 9th Ed., 1955.

(3) Seth, G., and Guthrie, D.: *Speech in Childhood; Its Development and Disorders.* London, Oxford University Press, 1935.

(4) Jespersen, O.: *Language; Its Nature, Development and Origin.* New York, Henry Holt, 1922.

(5) Carroll, J. B.: Language development. *Encyclopedia of Educational Research.* New York, The Macmillan Co., 1960, p. 744.

Chapter 3

FACTORS INFLUENCING THE NORMAL DEVELOPMENT OF SPEECH

I_T IS A fact that children vary a great deal in the onset of speech and in speech development. It is also a fact that adults vary greatly in speech effectiveness. What are some of the factors that influence the child's speech and language development? Authorities in the field have discussed the following influences on language development: sex, general intelligence, physical development, socio-economic environment, emotional factors, family constellation, and bilingualism. Each one of these influences on the child's development will be discussed.

SEX

A great deal has been written about the fact that girls talk earlier than boys. It has also been stressed that girls enjoy a much more rapid language growth than boys. Tests have shown that females begin with a greater vocabulary than males. Girls use words with greater fluency and accuracy. Karlin and Kennedy (1) quote Abt as finding that the usual onset of speech for boys is nineteen months, and for girls, eighteen months. McCarthy (2) says that at eighteen months 14 per cent of the responses made by boys and 38 per cent of those made by girls were comprehensible. She states, therefore, that intelligibility in speech occurs earlier in girls than in boys. Karlin believes that there may be some connection between earlier speech development in females and the fact that myelinization occurs earlier in girls than in boys.

On the other hand, authorities also point out that although speech development takes place earlier in girls than in boys, in the long run boys make up the lag at a later stage. They do not permanently stay behind females in language development. Templin (3) says, however, that "real deviations in language behavior are more frequent in boys than in girls."

26

GENERAL INTELLIGENCE

Intelligence is often measured by the child's knowledge of words and by his ability to use them. Many studies have shown a high correlation between non-verbal and verbal tests of abilities that are a measure of general intelligence. Thus, the measurement of vocabulary of younger children may well be one of the means of estimating their intelligence.

Simon (4) states that by eighteen months of age the child says some ten to twenty meaningful words. He will also continue his "little language" or jargon. By the age of two years, the child talks, making mistakes, but handles oral communication increasingly effectively. Van Riper (5) states that the idiot of three years of age has the language development of a child of one year. West (6) says that idiots never learn to speak. At any rate, the parent, the pediatrician, the psychologist, and the speech pathologist will all consider the possibility of intellectual handicap if by two and one-half to three years of age the child has not spoken in intelligible phrases. Intellectual handicap, however, is only one of many possible reasons for delay in language and speech development.

It must be observed that although there are many factors in his environment that will influence the child's language development, he is not a totally inactive part of his surroundings. His growth in the use of speech depends not only on the stimulus he receives from the external environment, but on the stimulus he receives from within. His growth depends on his own curiosity and his desire for learning about new objects and their names. This curiosity is stimulated by the child's native intelligence. The inquisitiveness of a child of two or three years of age has been commented on in an earlier chapter. His inner drive for giving things a name, coupled with his powers for listening, remembering, and repeating the new word, are largely a matter of intelligence. The child has a sharpening intelligence and he enjoys using it. If he does not understand a phenomenon in his surroundings or if he cannot name it, he has the initiative and the desire to find out about it. It is well to heed the words of Templin (3) who states that, "Intelligence is an important factor in the child's development of an appropriate use of words, but the fact that a child is not talking at an early age does not necessarily indicate lack of mental ability."

Gurren, as a result of having interviewed hundreds of parents and their children who had defective language development, notes that those children who are retarded intellectually suffer more from lack of vocabulary and use of language structure than from purely articulatory defects. In general, the per cent of articulatory defects in retardates is the same as in a group of non-retarded school children. The incidence of infantilisms is somewhat higher in the retarded group.

PHYSICAL DEVELOPMENT

The child's development in manual dexterity, walking, and in speech depends upon his physical maturation. If an infant is sickly, bedridden, or physically handicapped in any other way, his development of many skills will be retarded. Since speech development is stimulated by experiences, the physically handicapped child who cannot enjoy the play activities of the non-handicapped child, may not be stimulated to talk. The child whose vision and hearing have gained in acuity as a process of maturation will have more environmental experiences to aid in speech development.

Since language perception and speech motor centers are located in cortical areas that attain anatomical differentiation later than other motor centers, the element of time is an important factor in speech development. Speech, for example, requires finer coordination of small, delicately articulated muscles than does walking. The physical equipment for speech and the normal maturation of this equipment are essential to normal speech development.

SOCIO-ECONOMIC ENVIRONMENT

The fact that human beings vary a great deal both in speed of speech development in early childhood and in speech effectiveness in adult life is due in some measure to social and economic factors. Investigators show that children from more affluent homes have vocabularies about eight months in advance of those from poorer homes. In areas where there are wide differences in the economic status of groups, there are bound to be wide differences in vocabulary growth in children. On the other hand, in communities where there is a uniformly high standard of living and a high rate of literacy, there will be less marked differences in the language growth of children. One important leveling factor, however, in growth of vocabulary is the almost universal use of television in the United States. Children see and hear speech from this medium at a very early age. Television sets are to be found in the homes of the rich and poor alike.

EMOTIONAL FACTORS

Perhaps one of the most important environmental factors in development of speech is the emotional "atmosphere" in the home. Some parents are over-protective, others may be so preoccupied as to be uninterested in the child's language development. A child who is "babied" may obtain what he wants by pointing and making noises. There is no need for this child to talk. He does very well without speech. On the other hand, the child who is left to himself, who does not have the companionship of someone who will listen and respond to him, will have as little incentive to speak as the "spoiled" child.

Above all, a home in which there are frictions, quarrels, tensions, and emotional upsets is bound to have its effect on the child. The emotional atmosphere in the home influences the child. Some children react to tension by being insecure and frightened. These children often suffer serious effects on their speech development. Others may develop a speech defect such as stuttering as a result of nervous reactions on the part of the parents. Still others may be shy and withdrawn, with evidences of a dread of communication through speech. These speech difficulties are definite handicaps when the child becomes older and begins to play with others. They may act as serious deterrents to educational progress when the child is ready for school.

FAMILY CONSTELLATION

Children develop speech faster in homes where there is some response to their efforts to speak. It is true that at first the child's early babblings are for his own enjoyment, but he soon reacts to the responses he obtains from those in his environment.

The size of the family into which the child is born may influence the development of speech. Children copy their peers more readily than they imitate adults. The youngest child, if he has no handicaps, or if he is not "babied," will learn to speak more quickly than one who has no siblings.

Self-sufficient children develop speech more slowly than those who receive vocal reinforcement from the environment. Thus, it has been observed that twins develop speech more slowly than other children. Twins of above average intelligence, age seven, were observed by Gurren over a period of two years. They used the *idioglossia* characteristic of some twins who are so self-sufficient that they have no need to play with other children, nor to talk with adults. Their speech was completely unintelligible to their teacher, and to almost everyone in their environment. Their mother understood a few words here and there. It was obvious to Gurren that the boys were enjoying their secret form of communication, and that it would require a great deal of motivation to get them to talk in ordinary language. Following group speech therapy, it was decided that the boys should be placed in a school that housed a speech center. Here they receive speech instruction and stimulation from a specialist five times a week, whereas their former speech program provided for speech therapy once a week only. At the present time there is progress, although it is very slow. There is a great need for these bright boys to communicate on a level with their intellectual ability. As they mature, and as the parents provide stimulation in the home to carry on the work of the speech specialist in the school, it is presumed that these boys will abandon their immature attitude toward the outside world.

It has been observed that children brough up in institutions develop speech more slowly than those who live in a family environment. Templin (3) says, "One can interpret findings in the light of family constellation, but another legitimate way is that the amount and quality of talking in the child's environment is a factor to be considered in appraising language status. There is increasing evidence that increased language stimulation will increase the rate of language growth."

BILINGUALISM

The problem of bilingualism is prevalent in many large industrial cities. While it is desirable to speak more than one language well, and the time to learn language is at an early age, in many cases children of low economic level seldom learn the language of their parents well enough to speak it. Yet, the influence of the parents' language makes it difficult for the child to speak English fluently. Later, at school, he has difficulty not only with speech, but with reading and writing as well. In other words, many children in these circumstances, instead of being *bilingual* are actually *alingual.* They speak neither the language of their parents nor English fluently and effectively.

Gurren has observed many children who were born in this country but who heard another language at home, either from parents or grandparents. Many of them understand both English and the language of their parents. Their great lack is in the production of either language. By the time they reach school, they are somewhat behind the other children in vocabulary and in the use of characteristic English patterns. Their pronunciation is often foreign as well. This kind of difficulty is a definite handicap educationally and socially.

Gurren notes from observations of children born abroad that the first language a child learns to speak has deep roots. It is difficult for the child to give up his first language and to think in a new one. He identifies his first language with his home and his parents. For some time he finds it almost impossible to express himself in a strange tongue. However, the younger the child comes to this country, the easier it is for him to find his way in a new language. An adolescent student from a foreign country, after considerable instruction in English, still found it difficult to learn to think in the new language. He finally told Gurren that he must be nearing that goal because the night before he had "dreamed in English."

HEREDITY AND ENVIRONMENT

The relative importance of heredity and environment in the development of the child has long been a matter of discussion. As far as the development of speech is concerned, the child may inherit certain capacities and certain behavioral tendencies. First, the inherited intellectual capabilities will greatly influence his language development. Second, there are innate inherited tendencies to babble or to make sounds. This factor is essential to the development of speech.

On the other hand, it is necessary to point out that very early in the child's life the environment exercises a strong influence on his language development. After the earliest stages, the child "selects" his own speech models. Actually, there is no selection, since the imitation of the models is unconscious on the part of the child. He will copy the phonetic and syntactic patterns as well as the vocabulary of his environment. In an environment of low cultural level, the child will hear and use the vocabulary, grammar, and phonetic structure of his surroundings. He may have to relearn many aspects of the language when he enters school. On the other hand, the child who hears speech that is closer to that used in school, though he may not be brighter than a child from a lower cultural level, will begin school with an advantage because of his more skilled use of language.

In conclusion, the best situation is one in which the child is allowed to develop speech at his own rate with encouragement, but not insistence, from his family. A happy, normal child in a home in which he hears language reasonably well spoken will learn that pattern from his surroundings.

REFERENCES

(1) Karlin, I. W., and Kennedy, L.: Delay in Development of Speech. *Am. J. Dis. Child.*, 51:1138, May, 1936.

(2) McCarthy, D. A.: *Language Development of the Preschool Child.* Institute of Child Welfare Monograph Series, No. 4. Minneapolis, University of Minnesota Press, 1930.

(3) Templin, M.: *Panel Discussion on Childhood Aphasia.* Palo Alto, Stanford University Institute on Childhood Aphasia, September, 1960.

(4) Simon, C. T.: The Development of Speech. In Travis, L. E.: *Handbook of Speech Pathology.* New York, Appleton-Century-Crofts, 1957.
(5) Van Riper, C.: *Speech Correction; Principles and Methods.* New York, Prentice-Hall, 1963.
(6) West, R., Ansberry, M., and Carr, A.: *The Rehabilitation of Speech.* New York, Harper & Brothers, 1957.

Part II
THE MECHANISM FOR SPEECH PRODUCTION

Chapter 4

PERIPHERAL STRUCTURES
CONCERNED WITH SPEECH

Fʀᴏᴍ a phylogenetic point of view, speech is the newest of man's skills. For its normal development, one must have a normally functioning brain, normal peripheral anatomical structures used in speech, adequate hearing, and also a stimulating environment. An intact visual mechanism is also important.

The peripheral anatomical structures are not special organs set aside solely for speech. Speech has arrogated to itself structures such as the mouth, lungs and larynx that biologically perform more vital and quite different functions. The central nervous system acts as an integrator of these organs which are otherwise dissociated in function. It is only in the brain that certain areas have been developed whose function is predominantly concerned with speech.

Some authorities stress the idea that the function of the peripheral structures concerned with speech is basically biological, evolved for the preservation of the life of the individual. These investigators believe speech to be a borrowed function, utilizing the peripheral structures for its own purposes. Others believe that the peripheral structures have a dual function.

West states that articulation of speech may be as proper and natural a function of the mouth as chewing. Voice may be as genuine a basic function of the larynx as laryngeal constriction in straining or in lifting. Furthermore, listening to communication may be as fundamental a use of the ear as responding to the mating call in the forest.

The peripheral anatomical structures concerned with speech are so numerous and their arrangement so intricate and complex that for a detailed description of them, one has to consult textbooks of anatomy and physiology. For speech purposes, it will suffice to give a concise description of the anatomy and physiology of the systems from which the spoken word is fashioned.

First to be considered is the *respiratory* system. Air from the lungs is the initiating power from which the resonating and articulate sound of the voice is produced. Second is the *vocal* system. Voice, the fundamental note, is produced by the vibration of the vocal cords within the larynx. The third is the *resonating* system. Supraglottic structures resonate to the fundamental laryngeal tones and add specific qualities to them. Finally, one must study the *articulatory* system. Structures of the mouth such as the lips, teeth, gum ridge, tongue, hard and soft palates, and mandible shape the sounds transmitted to them into vowels and consonants.

RESPIRATORY SYSTEM
Anatomy of the Respiratory System

Respiration provides the air that will phonate, resonate, and provide the means for articulate sounds.

The *lungs* are the essential organ of respiration. They are situated in the *thorax* on either side of the *mediastinum.* The *thoracic cavity* is a closed cavity which changes constantly in size during respiration. The cavity is closed below by the *diaphragm* and above by the *scalene muscles* and the *fascia* of the neck. On the sides, front and back, the thoracic cavity is enclosed by *ribs, intercostal muscles, vertebrae,* the *sternum* and *ligaments.*

The thoracic cavity contains the two *pleural cavities,* each containing a lung. Each pleural cavity has a lining of serous membrane, the *pleura.* The layer lining the chest wall is called the *parietal pleura* and that over the lung the *visceral pleura.* Normally, the parietal pleura is not adherent to the visceral pleura. They are separated only by a potential pleural space containing pleural fluid for lubrication. The parietal pleura is well supplied with sensory nerve endings. These give rise to the sensation of pain in pleurisy.

The lungs in a healthy adult are spongy and completely fill the pleural cavity. The color of the lung of a baby is pink, owing to contained blood. In the adult, this color is marked by a mottled blue-gray color produced by inhaled particles of dust and soot which are permanently incorporated into lung tissue. The lung of an infant before he has breathed, is solid and sinks in water. After birth, respiration causes the lung to become spongy and filled with air, so that it no longer sinks. Complete opening of the air spaces of the lung is not attained until two to three weeks after birth.

The left lung has two lobes, an upper and a lower. The right lung has three: an upper, middle, and lower (see Figure 1). The right upper and middle lobes correspond to the left upper lobe. The right lung is wider and slightly larger than the left.

The *trachea* or windpipe splits at its lower end into two main *bronchi* (Fig. 2). As the bronchi pass into the substance of the lung, they subdivide into smaller and smaller divisions

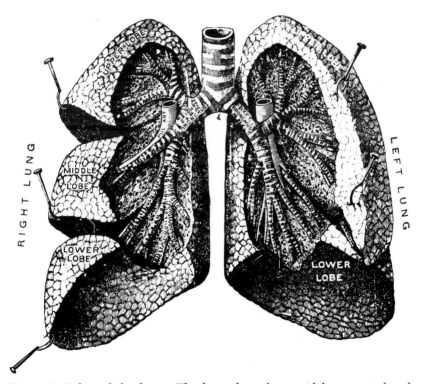

Figure 1. Lobes of the lungs. The lungs have been widely separated and tissue cut away to expose the bronchi and bronchioles. From Henry Gray's *Anatomy of the Human Body*, 27th Ed., edited by Charles Mayo Goss, 1959. Courtesy of Lea & Febiger, Philadelphia, Pennsylvania.

known as *bronchial tubes.* The bronchial tubes again divide into smaller and smaller passages which open into *alveolar ducts.*

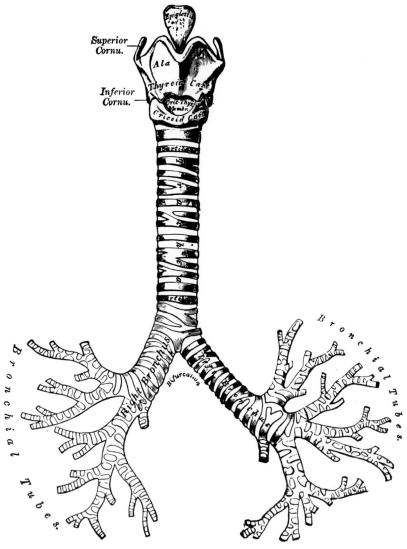

Figure 2. Front view showing bifurcation of trachea into bronchi and bronchial tubes. From Henry Gray's *Anatomy of the Human Body,* 27th Ed., edited by Charles Mayo Goss, 1959. Courtesy of Lea & Febiger, Philadelphia, Pennsylvania.

These ducts terminate into several *alveolar sacs* having numerous *alveoli*. The structure of the alveolar duct with its branching alveolar sacs can be likened to a bunch of grapes. The stem represents the alveolar duct; each cluster of grapes represents an alveolar sac; and each grape represents an alveolus.

Movements of Respiration

During inspiration, the diaphragm and external intercostal muscles contract due to impulses from the central nervous system by way of the *phrenic* and *intercostal nerves* (see Figure 3).

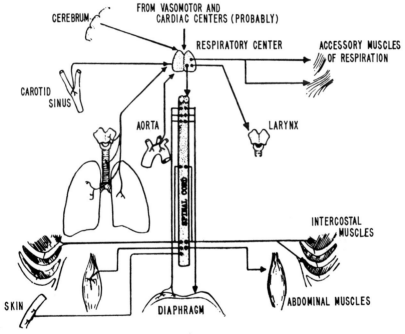

Figure 3. Diagram to illustrate the nervous control of respiration. From Charles Best and Norman Taylor's *The Physiological Basis of Medical Practice,* 7th Ed., 1961. Courtesy of The Williams & Wilkins Company, Baltimore, Maryland.

As the diaphragm contracts, its dome moves down and enlarges the thoracic cavity from top to bottom. The contraction of external intercostal muscles moves the ribs upward. This not only raises the sternum but moves it further from the spinal column, increasing the antero-posterior diameter of the chest. At the same time, the ribs are everted. The eversion increases the lateral diameter of the chest.

Since the lungs are connected with the outside air by conductive passages which are always open (nose, pharynx, larynx, trachea, and bronchi), air enters the lungs until the air pressure within them is equal to atmospheric pressure.

Respiration is the gaseous exchange between the organism and its environment. It consists primarily in the absorption of oxygen and the release of carbon dioxide. The transfer of oxygen and carbon dioxide between the outside air and the alveoli is referred to as "external" respiration. The transfer between the alveoli and body cells is called "internal" respiration.

Regulation of External Respiration

Respiration is rhythmic and ordinarily subconscious. The muscles of respiration are skeletal muscles. Unlike cardiac muscle, they have no inherent rhythmicity. In order to contract, they must have nerve stimulation. The normal activities of the individual create a widely fluctuating demand for oxygen. The respiratory center is exceedingly sensitive to this demand, largely because of an elaborate reflex adjustment. These reflex adjustments are made possible through *inspiratory* and *expiratory* *centers* as well as through the mechanism of the *Hering-Breuer reflex* which is described in the next section.

Respiratory Center

The *respiratory center* is a collection of nerve cells in the *medulla* which discharges impulses to the muscles of respiration (see Figure 4).

The *inspiratory center* occupies the rostral half or two-thirds of the *reticular formation,* overlying the *olivary nuclei* on both sides. When stimulated, a maximal coordinated inspiration results, involving both diaphragm and thorax.

The *expiratory center* or *inhibito-inspiratory center,* lies in the reticular formation dorsal to the inspiratory center. Stimulation within this area causes expiration.

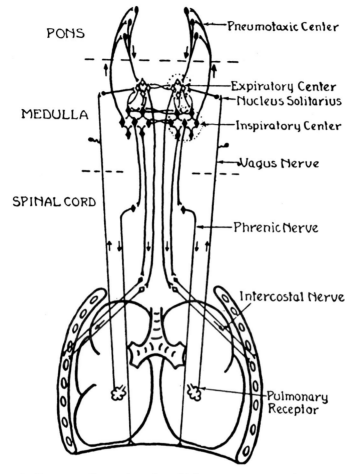

Figure 4. Diagram illustrating the chief nervous connections responsible for control of the respiratory rhythm. Inspiratory and expiratory centers in the medulla on the right side are surrounded by dotted circles. (After Pitts, slightly modified.) From Charles Best and Norman Taylor's *The Physiological Basis of Medical Practice*, 7th Ed., 1961. Courtesy of The Williams & Wilkins Company, Baltimore, Maryland.

Regular respirations, consisting of inspiration alternating with expiration, are induced by rhythmic stimulation of the inspiratory center. Expiration then occurs passively. The expiratory center is inactive in quiet breathing. When breathing is more active as in muscular exercise, the expiratory center also becomes active. It then sends out rhythmic impulses alternating with the inspiratory center. The expiratory muscles then contract. The respiratory center can also be stimulated or depressed by changes in the carbon dioxide and oxygen concentrations of the blood.

The Hering-Breuer Reflex

Inspiration and expiration are also regulated by a reflex first described by Hering and Breuer in 1868. These investigators demonstrated that inflation of the lungs arrested inspiration, expiration then ensuing. Likewise, deflation inhibited expiration and brought on inspiration.

The afferent component of this reflex consists of *vagus fibers* arising in lung tissue. The efferent path consists of both the phrenic nerve which innervates the diaphragm, and the intercostal nerves that innervate the intercostal muscles. The alveoli contain *stretch receptors*. Near the end of inspiration, the alveolar walls become stretched and this stimulates sensory nerve endings located in the walls. These impulses are transmitted via the vagus nerve to the inspiratory center and inhibit its activity. Similarly, retraction of the lungs during expiration sends a reflex impulse to inhibit the expiratory center.

BREATHING AND SPEECH

In normal quiet respiration, the inspiratory phase is about equal to the expiratory phase, though inspiration takes a little longer than expiration. In speech, the process is reversed. Expiration takes longer than inspiration. We can talk only on expired air. Although expiration is mainly a passive function, the diaphragm has a certain degree of muscle tonus. Therefore, on expiration the air is expelled from the lungs slowly, allowing a steady stream of air for speech purposes.

Many different systems of breathing and breath control for speech have been described and advocated. *Abdominal breathing* emphasizes predominantly the activity of the diaphragm. The *thoracic type* emphasizes the activity of the chest. The *medial type,* centering about the base of the sternum, emphasizes that breathing should be both diaphragmatic and thoracic. *Clavicular breathing* is upper chest breathing. In this method, the clavicles rise by the action of the neck muscles.

The current view is that speech may be just as effective whether one uses predominantly abdominal, thoracic or medial breathing. Clavicular type of breathing, however, should be avoided since it promotes tension in the region of the neck and throat, and will produce unsteadiness and tremulous expiration during speech.

In speech there is need for a somewhat prolonged, steady act of expiration. The less it interferes with normal respiration the better. In singing, breathing exercises are entirely directed toward expiration and its control.

THE VOCAL SYSTEM
Anatomy of the Larynx

The *larynx* is a short tube situated between the *trachea* and the *pharynx*. It is primarily a valvular mechanism leading into the trachea.

The larynx, or voice box, occupies a median, superficial position anteriorly in the neck. It is located opposite the fourth, fifth, and sixth cervical vertebrae. The upper part of the larynx communicates with the pharynx and is intimately attached to the *hyoid bone* and the *tongue.* The lower part is continuous with the trachea which also occupies a median position but is considerably deeper than the larynx (see Figure 5).

A man's larynx is about one-third larger than a woman's, which is about one-third larger than that of a child at birth. The larynx grows rapidly until the age of three years. At puberty, there is another period of rapid growth, especially in boys.

The larynx is suspended from the hyoid bone by the *hyothyroid membrane.* The hyoid bone is suspended from the tips of the *styloid processes* of the temporal bones by the *stylohyoid ligaments.* The hyoid, known as the *lingual bone,* has no direct connection with any other bone. It serves for the attachment of those muscles which move the tongue and aid in speaking and swallowing.

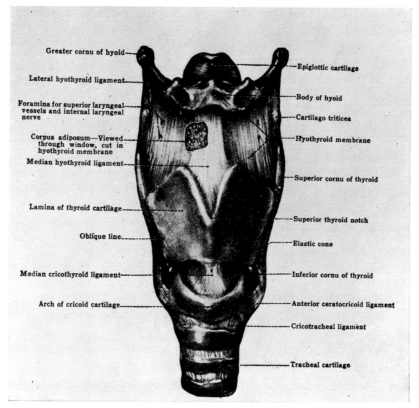

Figure 5. The laryngeal skeleton, as viewed from the ventral aspect. From Henry Morris' *Human Anatomy*, 11th Ed., edited by J. Parsons Schaeffer, 1953. Courtesy of Blakiston Div., McGraw-Hill Book Company, Inc., New York, New York.

Laryngeal Cartilages

The larynx is composed of *cartilages,* which are connected by ligaments and moved by numerous muscles. Of the nine cartilages of the larynx, there are three single cartilages and three paired cartilages in the laryngeal wall. The single cartilages are: *thyroid, cricoid,* and *epiglottis.* The paired cartilages are: *arytenoid, corniculate,* and *cuneiform* (see Figure 6).

The cartilages which are of most significance in voice production are the "shield like" thyroid cartilage, "ring like" cricoid cartilage, and the right and left arytenoid cartilages.

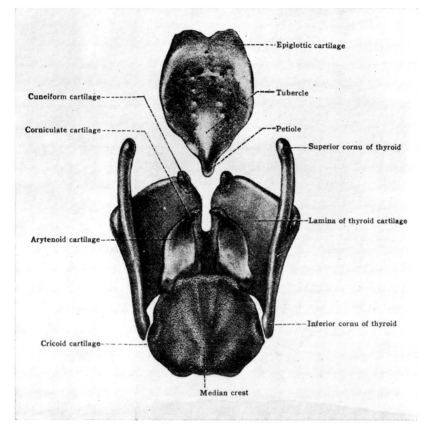

Figure 6. The cartilages of the larynx in their natural interrelationships, as viewed from the dorsal aspect. From Henry Morris' *Human Anatomy*, 11th Ed., edited by J. Parsons Schaeffer, 1953. Courtesy of Blakiston Div., McGraw-Hill Book Company, Inc., New York, New York.

The thyroid cartilage is the largest of these cartilages. It forms the front of the voice box. It is composed of two laminae which are widely separated posteriorly, but are fused anteriorly where they form the laryngeal prominence known as the "Adam's apple." The upper borders of the laminae diverge to produce a deep, narrow V-shaped notch, the *thyroid notch,* situated just above the laryngeal prominence. The posterior border of each lamina is prolonged to form the *superior* and *inferior cornua* or horns. The upper border of the thyroid cartilage is attached to the hyoid bone by a dense fibrous sheet, the hyothyroid membrane. Its posterior margins are thickened to form the *lateral hyothyroid ligaments,* uniting with the superior cornua of the thyroid cartilage. The inferior cornua articulate with the arytenoid cartilage.

The cricoid cartilage is the only complete ring of the larynx. It is situated between the thyroid cartilage above and the first tracheal ring below. It consists of a lamina posteriorly and an arch anteriorly.

The two arytenoid cartilages are small triangular pyramids located in the posterior section of the larynx.

The right and left corniculate cartilages are attached to the apices of the arytenoid cartilages. The right and left cuneiform cartilages are small, yellow, rod-shaped pieces of cartilage in the *aryepiglottic folds,* which are membranes stretching between the epiglottis above and the arytenoids below. They are not always present.

Each lateral superior border of the cricoid cartilage bears a small facet against which the concave facet of each arytenoid base articulates. On the lateral border of the cricoid lamina, at its junction with the arch, is a facet for articulation with the inferior cornu of the thyroid cartilage. These two pairs of facets are the only articular surfaces of the larynx.

The epiglottis is a thin leaf-like cartilage. It is situated behind the hyoid bone and the base of the tongue. The stem of the leaf, or *petiole,* is attached to the inner surface of the thyroid by the *thyroepiglottic ligament.* The posterior laryngeal surface presents a convexity, the *epiglottic tubercle,* which is visible on laryngoscopic examination. The anterior surface extends by means of ligaments to the sides and root of the tongue. The epiglottis serves to deflect food to the esophagus. It may also add to resonance by producing changes in size of the laryngeal cavity.

The Vocal Cords or Folds

The *vocal cords* are also called folds or bands. The term folds is descriptive since the structures are prominent folds which project from the inner wall of the larynx (see Figures 7 and 8). During phonation, the vocal cords are in approximation.

The vocal cords are divided into the *true* and *false vocal cords.*

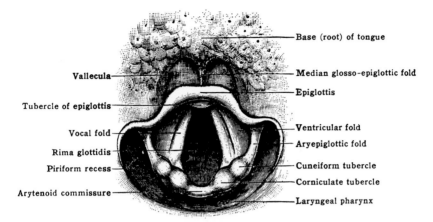

Figure 7. View of interior of larynx as seen from above during inspiration. From Henry Morris' *Human Anatomy,* 11th Ed., edited by J. Parsons Schaeffer, 1953. Courtesy of Blakiston Div., McGraw-Hill Book Company, Inc., New York, New York.

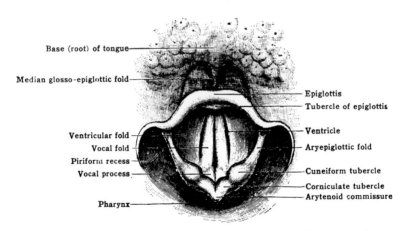

Figure 8. View of interior of larynx as seen from above during vocalization. From Henry Morris' *Human Anatomy,* 11th Ed., edited by J. Parsons Schaeffer, 1953. Courtesy of Blakiston Div., McGraw-Hill Book Company, Inc., New York, New York.

The true vocal cords represent the thickened upper margin of the cricothyroid membrane. They are pearly white in color and are composed of yellow elastic tissue. Subjacent to the elastic edge of the vocal cord is the thyroarytenoid muscle. Fibers of this muscle constitute the *aryvocalis muscle* which is attached to the cord. The vocal cord extends from the thyroid cartilage, near the midline, to the vocal process and part of the body of the arytenoid. The function of the vocal cords is production of sound.

Between the true vocal cords is a narrow chink, the *rima glottidis*. Just above the true vocal cords are the paired ventricular or false vocal cords. They are rounded, fleshy, mucous folds representing the inferior free margins of the quadrangular membrane. They resemble in appearance the true vocal cords and are attached posteriorly to the arytenoids. The space between the entrance to the larynx above and the ventricular folds below is known as the *vestibule*. The space between the ventricular folds and the vocal cords is known as the *ventricle*.

The false vocal cords are part of the protective mechanism by which the airway is closed against the entry of food or foreign bodies.

The mucous membrane of the larynx is furnished with numerous mucous secreting glands. These glands are also found in the false vocal cords as well as in front of the arytenoid cartilages (*arytenoid glands*). None are found on the free edges of the true vocal cords. The glands, in addition to supplying moisture to the laryngeal cavity, also supply the mucous necessary to lubricate the true vocal cords.

Intrinsic Muscles of the Larynx

There are five intrinsic muscles of the larynx (see Figure 9).

1. Paired *lateral cricoarytenoid muscles,* one on each side, are adductors. Their action brings the vocal cords parallel and approximates them.
2. The unpaired *arytenoid muscle* is also an adductor. It pulls the arytenoid processes together and closes the glottis, especially the back part.
3. Paired *thyroarytenoid muscles* are also adductors. Fibers of these muscles are in the substance of the vocal cords. Contraction of these muscles, together with the arytenoid, closes the glottis. They also impart to the edges of the vocal cords varying degrees of hardness or elasticity.

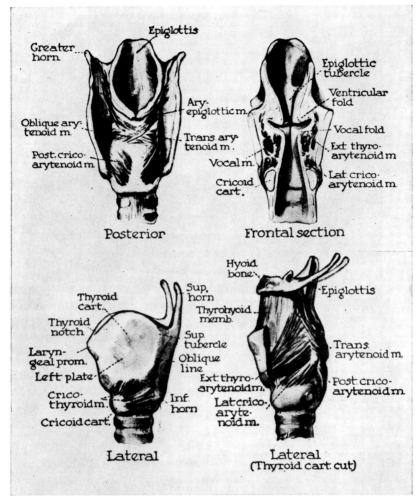

Figure 9. The intrinsic muscles of the larynx; four views are shown. From Philip Thorek's *Anatomy in Surgery*, 2nd Ed., 1962. Courtesy of the J. B. Lippincott Company, Philadelphia, Pennsylvania.

4. Paired *cricothyroid muscles* produce tension on the vocal cords and aid phonation.
5. Paired *posterior cricoarytenoids* are abductors. They are the most powerful of the laryngeal muscles and are the only ones that open the glottis.

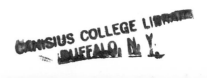

The inferior laryngeal nerve supplies all the muscles of the larynx except the cricothyroid which is supplied by the superior laryngeal nerve.

MECHANISM OF VOICE PRODUCTION (PHONATION)

Phonetics is the science of speech sounds. It is the study of sound formation by the speech organs and their perception by the ear.

Normal voice is due to the vibration of the vocal cords brought about by a column of expired air from the lungs. The action of the vocal cords sets up a complex motion in the adjacent air. The moving air current produces a fundamental tone and a large number of overtones. This sound is called "cord tone." This spectrum is then modified by passage through the resonators in the supraglottic cavities (*vocal resonance theory*).

The action of the vocal cords has been studied by means of inspection, high speed motion photography, and by stroboscopic examination. In general, results indicate that movements of the vocal cords are most complex at low frequencies and become simpler as the frequency and tone are raised. At extremely high frequencies, only the edges of the vocal cords adjacent to the glottis are seen to vibrate. There is still no definite evidence of what specific action of the vocal cords is responsible for the production of sound.

THEORIES OF VOICE PRODUCTION

Various theories of voice production have been postulated. Three hypotheses will be discussed.

Vibratory String Theory

The vibratory string theory states that just prior to speaking, the vocal cords are approximated by the adductor muscles and thrown into vibration by the expiratory blast of air from the lungs. The resulting vibration produces a note, the pitch of which varies according to the tension and shape of the vocal cords. The vocal cords may be vibrated in whole, producing the fundamental tone, or in part, which produces the overtones. When air pressure is blown from below, the margins of the cords separate so as to leave a slit-like aperture. Then by recoil, the cords meet again at their margin. The phases of opening and closing succeed one another with great rapidity and the vibrations of the vocal cords produce a vocal note.

Aerodynamic (Tonic) Theory

The aerodynamic or tonic theory of voice production postulates that when sufficient pressure is built up below the glottis by the air stream from the lungs, the adducted vocal cords are blown apart. This action releases small puffs of air. The puffs of air, resulting from alternating opening and closing of the cords, produce sound. The number of air puffs that are released per second determines the pitch of the sound produced.

Neurochronaxic (Clonic) Theory

The neurochronaxic or clonic theory states that the vocal cords are capable of vibrating independently of the air stream. The rhythmic impulses passing down the inferior laryngeal nerve from the cerebrum, stimulate fibers of the thyroarytenoid muscles to corresponding rhythmic contractions. The rate of contraction determines the pitch of the sounds produced. Air is necessary, however, for the transmission of the sound waves. The origin of the vibration is in the rhythmic activity of the brain cells governing the inferior laryngeal nerve fibers. In the previous theories, the blast of expired air from the lungs is thought to initiate activity by the vocal cords. In the neurochronaxic theory, however, nervous stimulation from the cerebrum is thought to initiate vibrations in the cords.

THE RESONATING SYSTEM

Physics defines resonance as prolongation or modification of a sound by means of transmission of sympathetic vibrations of one sounding body to another. The quality of the sound can be modified in a great variety of ways.

The fundamental tone produced by the vocal cords is modified by the resounding bodies. The personal characteristic of an individual's voice depends upon the type of resonators he possesses.

The resonators give the voice its individual timbre and permit the recognition of each person's voice.

Anatomy and Physiology of the Resonators

The human resonators consist of the *oral cavity*, the *pharynx*, the *hard palate*, and the *nasal passages*. For practical purposes, the most important are the cavities of the mouth and pharynx.

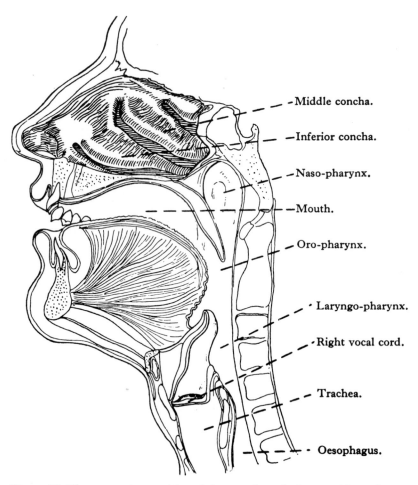

Figure 10. The resonating cavities of the mouth and pharynx. From George Seth and Douglas Guthrie's *Speech in Childhood*, 1935. Courtesy of Oxford University Press, London, England.

These resonators are dynamic. Their shape changes as they adapt themselves to the pronunciation of vowels and consonants needed for articulation of words.

The pharynx consists of three parts: *nasopharynx, oropharynx,* and *laryngopharynx* (see Figure 10). The upper part, nasopharynx, is posterior to the nasal cavities. The middle part, oropharynx, lies posterior to the mouth and is the only part visible on looking into the mouth. The inferior portion, laryngopharynx, is located behind the larynx and is continuous with the esophagus. The soft palate is closely associated with the function of the pharynx (Fig. 11). When the soft palate is raised, it shuts off the nasopharynx from the lower pharynx and from the mouth. The closure may be assisted by the protrusion forward of *Passavant's cushion,* resulting from a contraction of fibers of the palatopharyngeal muscle (see Figure 12). This closure directs the exhaled air into the oral cavity during the production of all English sounds except the nasal consonants *m, n, ng.*

Resonance may also be influenced by the *cul-de-sac principle.* Cul-de-sac is a tube or cavity, open at one end and connected to a resonator. In nasal sounds, when the oral passageway to the outer air is occluded, as it is with *m, n,* and *ng,* and the sound waves are emitted through the nasal fossae, the mouth acts as the cul-de-sac. In oral sounds, the nose becomes the cul-de-sac. In either case, the cul-de-sac principle is a contributory factor toward resonance in speech.

The mouth is one of the most important resonators since it is an open cavity with its size and shape subject to wide modifications. In addition, the mouth alone is the apparatus for articulation.

The nose, through its nasal passages, adds normal nasal resonance. However, it is less selective, since unlike the mouth and pharynx, it is not adaptable to dimensional changes.

It is still a debatable question as to whether the *paranasal sinuses* contribute to resonance in speech. It is a fact, however, that pathology of the paranasal sinuses may change voice quality.

The resonators add carrying power to the voice. They also influence the overtones of the voice. This gives the voice its individual timbre and permits the recognition of each person as

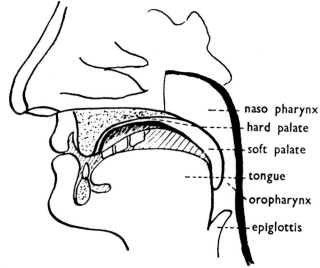

Figure 11. Soft palate in a resting condition. Air passing through the nose. From Muriel E. Morley's *Cleft Palate and Speech*, 5th Ed., 1962. Courtesy of E. & S. Livingstone Ltd., Edinburgh, Scotland.

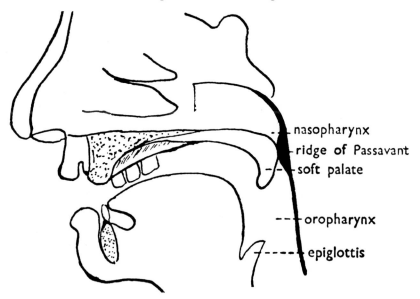

Figure 12. Soft palate raised. Palatopharyngeal sphincter closed. Air is passing through the mouth. From Muriel E. Morley's *Cleft Palate and Speech*, 5th Ed., 1962. Courtesy of E. & S. Livingstone Ltd., Edinburgh, Scotland.

he speaks. Thus, it is possible to distinguish the voice of a tenor from that of a baritone even when both sing the same note.

THE ARTICULATORY SYSTEM

Good articulation is defined as the act of pronouncing sounds and words distinctly. Articulation consists of highly complex movements of the *tongue, lips, teeth, jaw,* and *palate,* which constantly vary the size and shape of the oral and nasopharyngeal resonating cavities. Articulation is also a matter of conversion of kinetic energy of the breath stream into speech sounds.

The *mouth* alone is the place of articulation. The cavity of the mouth consists of its *vestibule* and the cavity proper, partially separated by the gums and teeth. The *orbicularis oris muscle* forms the foundation of the *lips.* The *buccinator* forms the foundation of the *cheeks.* In addition to the lips, the structures within the mouth are the actual articulators. These are the *tongue, hard* and *soft palate, teeth,* and *jaw.* Posteriorly, the cavity of the mouth opens into the pharynx.

Nerve Supply of the Articulators

The muscles of the face and lips are innervated by the *facial nerve,* the seventh cranial nerve. The jaw is innervated by the *trigeminal* or fifth cranial nerve. The jaw is capable of more rapid movement than the lips and at the same time, carries the lips along with it. The tongue is innervated by the *hypoglossal* or twelfth cranial nerve. The tongue is the most mobile of the articulators.

Movement of the Articulators

Articulation consists of highly complex movements of the mobile parts such as the tongue, lips, and soft palate in relation to the fixed parts such as the teeth, upper gums, and hard palate. Movements of the jaw exercise a great influence upon articulation. The movements of the articulators constantly vary the size and shape of the resonating cavities. Ideally, there is a specific position for each articulator in the production of each sound. Actually, however, isolated positions for the articulators are not fixed entities. Different sounds can be elicited by the same articulators and two persons can produce a perfectly good sound with different positioning of the articulators.

The tongue, especially its tip, is the fastest articulator. From time immemorial, the tongue has been regarded as the chief organ of speech. It is also used for mastication and deglutition. The tongue is a muscular organ consisting of intrinsic and extrinsic muscles. The form and position of the tongue is altered by its muscular contraction.

The cheeks and lips are important articulators. They play a part in facial expression. In trained subjects, the meaning of speech may be appreciated by the visual interpretation gained from lip or face reading just as readily as by picking up the sound of speech by the ear. The movements of articulation are very important to speech production. They convey meaning, as opposed to emotional quality, to the spoken word.

METHODS OF ARTICULATION FOR LINGUISTIC SOUNDS

Gurren, in Table IV, summarizes the five chief ways in which the various mouth components articulate to produce the consonants. First, there are the *plosives* or *stops*. The sounds *b*, *d*, and *g* are examples. Here, the breath stream is completely stopped in the formation of these sounds. Secondly, there are the *fricatives* or *continuants*. For example, a narrow slit or groove is formed for the air in the production of the sounds *th* and *sh*. The *lateral* type is exhibited by the articulation in forming the sound *l*. Here, the sound front is prevented from going through the middle of the mouth. It passes out around one or both sides of the mouth. In the fourth or *nasal* type of articulation, the air column vibrating with the vocal tone, passes out through the nasal cavity while the articulatory surfaces of the oral cavity are approximated. This method is responsible for the production of *m*, *n*, and *ng*. The last type is the *semivowel*, of which the sounds *w* and *r* are examples.

In the case of consonants, there is some obstacle to the free exit of air from the oral cavity. In the articulation of vowels and semivowels, the tongue assumes the appropriate position and the sound wave passes freely out of the oral cavity. In the case of some vowels, such as *o*, the lips are rounded.

TABLE IV

ENGLISH CONSONANTS

POINTS OF ARTICULATION

MANNER OF ARTICULATION	Lips	Upper Teeth and Lower Lip	Upper Teeth	Upper Gum Ridge	Front Palate	Soft Palate
Stops or Plosives	p b			t d		k g
Continuants or Fricatives		f v	θ ð	s z / ʃ ʒ		
*Vowel-like Consonants	ʍ w			l	ɹ j	
**Affricated Consonants				tʃ dʒ		
Nasals	m			n		ŋ

*1. These consonants take the place of a vowel in a syllable, as in little lɪtl. The nasals m and n may also take the place of a vowel in a syllable, as in nation neɪʃn, and chasm kæzm.

**2. These are composed of two consonants, the first a stop; the second, a continuant. The word church tʃɝ·tʃ begins and ends with the affricated sound tʃ. The word judge begins and ends with the affricated consonant dʒ, dʒʌdʒ.

3. The sound h is formed by forcing air through the glottis.

Note: Letters printed in dark type indicate voiced sounds. Letters in light type indicate voiceless sounds.

Table IV. The English consonants showing point and manner of articulation, written in the International Phonetic Alphabet (after Gurren).

SUMMARY

There is a great similarity between voice production and production of tone in musical instruments. Three factors operate in both cases. First, there is a force that puts a vibrating mechanism into action. Second, there is the vibrating mechanism itself. And last, there are resonators that modify certain vibrations. In the human voice, the force is given by the blast of expired air sent through the trachea by the lungs. The true vocal cords form the vibratory mechanism. The resonators are made up of the supraglottic cavities, consisting of the upper larynx, pharynx, nose, and mouth.

The intensity or loudness of a voice is directly proportional to the amplitude of the vibrations of the true vocal cords. The vibrations increase with the force of expiration. Loudness of voice is measured in decibels. There is approximately a 100 decibel difference between the softest whisper and the loudest cry. In ordinary conversation, loudness of voice varies between forty and sixty decibels.

Chapter 5

CENTRAL STRUCTURES
CONCERNED WITH SPEECH

THE PERIPHERAL structures used in speech are mediated by muscular activity of the various systems described in the previous chapter. Speech involves a delicate coordination of respiration, phonation, resonance, and articulation. These activities not only have to be coordinated, but some of the functions must be modified. For example, the expiratory phase of respiration frequently has to be prolonged. Also, rhythm and precision of timing have to be established. The central nervous system is the integrator which combines into a functional whole all these semi-independent activities.

The highest development of language occurs in man. Man's speech results from evolutionary changes in the brain. The two principal factors leading to human speech development are: first, the great increase in the size of the brain in comparison to the rest of the body and second, the great increase in size and complexity of the cerebral hemispheres.

The terms speech and language frequently are used interchangeably. To be precise, however, the two are not synonymous. Speech consists of spoken words and reflects arbitrary audible symbols. It is the verbal means of communication and may be regarded both as a tool and as a manifestation of the higher function of language. Language is an enormously complicated process centered in the cerebral cortex. In its broadcast sense, language signifies the elaboration of thoughts and ideas. It also reflects the total personality of the individual. Fully developed, speech and language are at once the expression and the means of conducting mental processes which are beyond the reach of even the great apes.

STRUCTURE OF NERVOUS TISSUE

The structural unit of the nervous system is the *neuron,* too small to be seen with the naked eye. A typical neuron is multipolar and consists of a *cell body* with a single *axon* and several branched processes, known as *dendrites* (see Figure 13). The axon breaks up into many terminal subdivisions. Dendrites are at the opposite pole of the cell from the axon. The nerve impulse travels from the dendrites through the cell body and then along

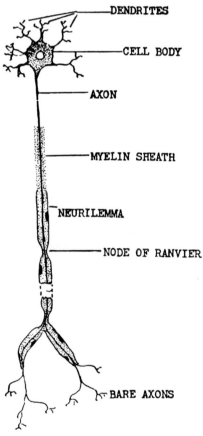

Figure 13. A diagram of the neuron showing its component structures. From Charles Best and Norman Taylor's *The Physiological Basis of Medical Practice,* 7th Ed., 1961. Courtesy of The Williams & Wilkins Company, Baltimore, Maryland.

the axon. Nerve cells are contiguous but not continuous. They are separated by a space, the *synaptic junction.* Transmission of nerve impulses from one nerve to another takes place at the synaptic junctions. Synapses allow impulses to travel in one direction only through the neuron. Connections are therefore never established between the dendrites of one neuron and those of another. Neurons which connect with sensory organs are termed *sensory neurons* and those whose axons terminate in muscles or glands are *motor neurons.* The neurons of the brain are *association neurons,* forming functional links between neuronal systems. The entire central nervous system is composed of billions of neurons as well as *glial supporting tissue.*

A nerve fiber is the axon of a nerve cell and may be short or several feet long, depending on its location and function. Nerve fibers usually have protective sheaths. There are two of these coverings for the nerve fibers: the *myelin sheath or medullary sheath* wrapped around the axons and the *neurilemma or sheath of Schwann,* which encloses the myelin sheath (see Figure 13). The myelin sheath is a lipoidal substance which gives the nerve a whitish appearance. The myelin sheath in a peripheral nerve has interruptions or constrictions along its course. These constrictions are called *nodes of Ranvier* (see Figure 13). The axon, however, runs without interruption through the nodes. The neurilemma or sheath of Schwann is a thin cellular membrane which encloses the myelin sheath. On myelinated nerves, there is a neurilemma cell for each internodal segment between nodes of Ranvier.

Nerve Fibers

Nerve fibers are of two types, *myelinated* and *non-myelinated.* The presence or absence of the myelin sheath determines whether nervous tissue is classified as *white matter* or *gray matter.* Aggregates of nerve fibers possessing myelin sheaths are called white matter. Accumulations of fibers in the brain without myelin are called gray matter. The bodies of the nerve cells lie within this gray matter of the central nervous system or in outlying *ganglia.*

All nerve fibers may be divided into four classes. First, naked axons without a sheath of any kind form the gray substance of the central nervous system. Second, non-medullated or gray fibers with a neurilemma sheath surrounding the axon are found in the autonomic nervous system and in afferent fibers of the cerebrospinal nerves. Third, myelinated or white fibers without a neurilemma sheath compose the white substance of the brain and spinal cord. Fourth, myelinated or white fibers with a neurilemma sheath make up the bulk of the cerebrospinal nerves.

Nerve fibers are also divided into *projection fibers, association fibers,* and *commisural fibers.* Projection fibers connect the brain with the spinal cord and are divided into descending and ascending groups, according to whether they conduct impulses to or from the cerebral cortex. The association fibers connect different structures in the same hemisphere. The commisural fibers connect the two halves of the brain.

THE BRAIN

During the process of evolution from fish to man, the *forebrain,* which was chiefly the seat of olfactory sensation, has become the

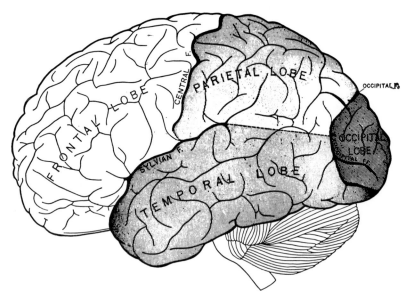

Figure 14. Principal fissures and lobes of the cerebrum viewed laterally. From Henry Gray's *Anatomy of the Human Body,* 27th Ed., edited by Charles Mayo Goss, 1959. Courtesy of Lea & Febiger, Philadelphia, Pennsylvania.

seat of all sensations. Its surface has become deeply convoluted to increase the surface area of the *cortex,* or *neopallium*. It has become the seat of volition, concept formation, purposeful action, speech, and personality.

The brain is lodged within the bony skull which serves as its protection. The brain has three *meningeal coverings: pia mater, arachnoid,* and *dura mater*. The thin and delicate pia is closely applied to the cortex. The arachnoid is a thin meshwork between pia and dura. The dura is tough and fibrous and is divided into two layers. The outer layer of the dura forms the *periosteum* of the skull. The inner layer forms the outer layer of the meninges. The dura also forms four processes: the *falx cerebri* which descends in the longitudinal fissure between the two hemispheres; the *tentorium cerebelli* which lies between the cerebellum and the occipital lobes; the *falx cerebelli;* and the *diaphragma sellae* which roofs in the *sella turcica* and almost completely covers the *hypophysis*.

CEREBRAL HEMISPHERES

The longitudinal fissure, containing the falx cerebri, partially divides the brain into two halves, forming the *cerebral hemispheres*. In the depth of the fissure, the hemispheres are united to each other by an extensive white commisural structure, the *corpus callosum*.

Each cerebral hemisphere is divided into lobes by various fissures (see Figure 14). The *Sylvian fissure* separates the *temporal lobe* below from the *frontal* and *parietal lobes* above. The *central sulcus* or *fissure of Rolando* forms the boundary between the frontal and parietal lobes. The *parieto-occipital fissure* is located between the *parietal* and *occipital lobes*. Thus, the fissures divide the cortex into frontal, parietal, occipital, and temporal lobes. The fissures of Sylvius and Rolando separate the anterior or motor cortex from the posterior or sensory cortex.

The *Island of Reil (Insula)* or *central lobe,* lies deep in the Sylvian fissure and is covered by the frontal and temporal lobes.

Basal Ganglia

The gray matter of the cerebrum, where the nerve cells are massed, forms the outer layer of the cortex, the extent of which is multiplied many times by the surface foldings. The interior of the brain is composed of white matter. Imbedded in the white matter of the cerebral hemispheres are masses of gray matter known as the *basal ganglia.* The basal ganglia consist of the *corpus striatum, amygdaloid nucleus,* and *claustrum.*

The corpus striatum is incompletely divided into two parts, the *caudate* and *lentiform nuclei.* The tail of the caudate nucleus

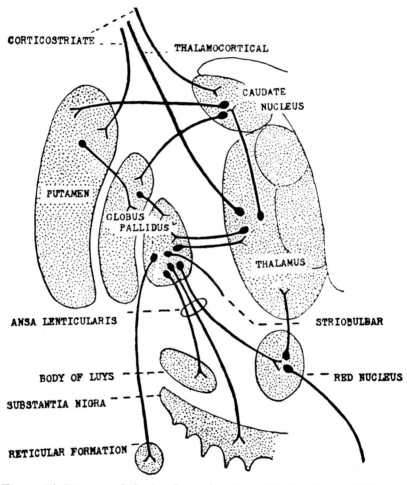

Figure 15. Diagram of the basal ganglia. From Charles Best and Norman Taylor's *The Physiological Basis of Medical Practice,* 7th Ed., 1961. Courtesy of The Williams & Wilkins Company, Baltimore, Maryland.

ends in the amygdaloid nucleus. The lentiform nucleus is divided into two parts. The smaller medial portion is yellowish in color and is named *globus pallidus*. The larger lateral portion is reddish in color and is named *putamen* (see Figure 15). Compressed between the lentiform nucleus laterally and the caudate nucleus and *thalamus* medially, is a group of ascending and descending projection fibers known as the *internal capsule*. The internal capsule is one of the most important groups of projection fibers. On the temporal side of the lentiform nucleus is a narrow band of white matter known as the *external capsule*. Lateral to the external capsule is an elongated island of gray matter known as the claustrum.

Physiologically, the basal ganglia control cortical activity at a higher level. They help control muscle tone. The clinically recognized pathological syndromes of the basal ganglia are of two main types: first, *Parkinson's Disease* or *paralysis agitans* characterized by coarse tremors and muscular rigidity, and second, involuntary movements of *athetosis* and *chorea*.

The thalamus is a mass of gray matter medial to the corpus striatum. It is a relay station for sensory impulses on their way from the periphery to the sensory areas of the cerebral cortex. Circumscribed lesions of the thalamus cause impairment of the sensations of pain, temperature, and touch.

Cerebellum

The *cerebellum* lies behind the *pons* and *medulla*. It lies beneath the occipital lobes of the cerebrum, from which it is separated by a process of dura mater called the *tentorium cerebelli*.

The cerebellum consists of a median portion called the *vermis* and *two cerebellar hemispheres* (see Figure 16). The cerebellar hemispheres expand laterally from the vermis and hug the sides of the medulla and pons.

Functionally, the cerebellum is concerned with the control of tonus and coordination of voluntary muscles. Its function is intimately related to posture, the maintenance of equilibrium, and the performance of habitual and practiced movements.

Lesions of the cerebellum, especially the vermis, will produce disturbances of speech due to *asynergia* of the muscles of phona-

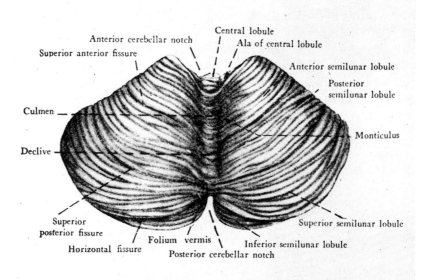

Figure 16. Upper surface of cerebellum. From Henry Morris' *Human Anatomy,* 11th Ed., edited by J. Parsons Schaeffer, 1953. Courtesy of Blakiston Div., McGraw-Hill Book Company, Inc., New York, New York.

tion and articulation. The speech abnormality may be drawling, jerky, scanning, or explosive in type.

CYTOARCHITECTURE OF THE CEREBRAL CORTEX

There are differences of opinion as to the specificity of function of certain areas of the brain. Some hold that there is pinpoint specificity and that brain function, including that of speech, is localized in circumscribed areas called centers. Others doubt this specialization and postulate that speech is the function of the entire cortex.

The term brain center has been more clearly defined by Nielsen (1). He points out that the word "center" does not mean a delimited cortical zone with *independent* functional capacity, but rather an anatomically delimited zone which is *essential* to a certain function. The term center will be used in the latter sense only, in this book.

Head (2), in his studies of aphasia, discards the concept of centers for the localization of speech. Nevertheless, he states that regions do exist in the cortex "where the progress of some mode of action can be reinforced, deviated, or inhibited." Perhaps a still better term would be "areas" in the brain where lesions produce disturbances of language.

The cerebral cortex has been subdivided into *cytoarchitectonic areas (Brodman's areas)*, based on microscopic studies. The differences in cytoarchitecture between two areas are not limited to a single layer, but usually extend to several. Brodman mapped out forty-seven areas. Only some of these will be enumerated, especially those concerned with speech (see Figure 17).

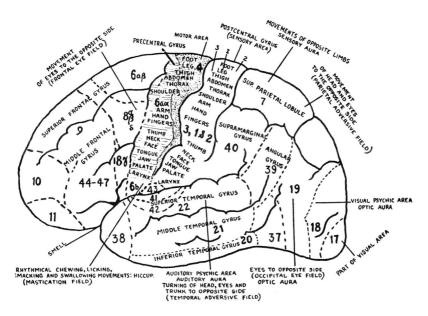

Figure 17. The cortex of the lateral surface of the cerebral hemisphere showing Brodman's areas. From Charles Best and Norman Taylor's *The Physiological Basis of Medical Practice*, 7th Ed., 1961. Courtesy of The Williams & Wilkins Company, Baltimore, Maryland.

The central sulcus or fissure of Rolando divides the more anteriorly placed *motor cortex, area 4,* from the posteriorly placed *sensory areas* of *3, 1,* and *2.* The frontal or motor areas are therefore divided from the parietal or sensory areas.

The normal activity of the central nervous system depends upon the interaction of sensory and motor systems. The sensory, or receptive component of speech, consists of comprehending spoken or written language, i.e., spoken words or written symbols. The motor, or expressive component of speech, consists in the ability to utter words or to write symbols.

The *auditory word area* for the comprehension of spoken language is in the *superior temporal gyrus*. It comprises *Wernicke's area, areas 41* and *42*. There is evidence that the adjoining portion of *area 22* subserves the same function. *Area 37* is the *language formulation area* where *engrams* are laid down for the proper arrangement of words into sentences. *Area 17* is the *primary visual center. Areas 18* and *19* are the *secondary visual centers* concerned with recognition of objects but no symbols. *Area 39* is the *visual word area* located in the *angular gyrus*. The visual areas of 17, 18, and 19 lie in the cortex of the occipital lobe. The *motor or expressive area* of speech is known as *Broca's area*. It is located at the posterior end of the inferior frontal convolution in the frontal lobe. Broca's area develops later than the other motor centers. Not until seventeen months after birth does it reach that degree of anatomical differentiation that can be observed in the other motor centers by the eleventh month. Broca's region is not the direct cortical representation of the muscles of speech, but lies just anterior to them. Fulton states that Broca's area has a characteristic cytoarchitecture even in monkeys and is possibly a development of that portion of *area 6* from which vocalization can be produced by stimulation in monkeys.

The *writing area* is part of the *chirokinesthetic area* and is situated above Broca's area. It is probably a part of the psychomotor area for the upper extremity.

Two conclusions can be drawn from the above localization of speech areas in the cortex. First, the sensory or receptive areas for speech are localized in the posterior part of the cerebral cortex, while the motor areas are primarily associated with the anterior cortex. Second, the areas of the cortex concerned with the reception and understanding of speech are much larger than those occupied with its expression.

CORTICAL AREAS CONCERNED WITH SPEECH

From a review of the above-mentioned cortical areas concerned with speech, one becomes aware that there is no single speech center in the brain with independent function. Instead, there are a number of anatomically delimited zones, each contributing to the total function of speech.

In the development of speech, associations are made between the sensory and motor areas outlined above. The child's first goal in language development is to form associations between verbal sounds, words, and their meanings. The child must first hear language for a certain period of time in order for the symbols to acquire their characteristic meaning. After hearing and understanding spoken words, he begins to talk himself. The sequence of events is as follows: reception of language, inner language, expression of language. The recognition of different sounds and the ability to reproduce them is a *sine qua non* of language. The child then learns to understand, recall, and reproduce the words that are applied to specific objects or activities. By the age of three, the child speaks in complete phrases or in short sentences which are grammatically correct. By the age of four or five, he can use several sentences to tell a story or carry on a conversation on a single subject. Thus, the division of the cortex into areas with different functions has not only anatomical importance, but physiological and, as will be seen later, pathological significance.

CEREBRAL DOMINANCE

A distinct attribute of the human brain is the dominance of one cerebral hemisphere over the other in the performance of language function. The left cerebral hemisphere is known as the dominant hemisphere in right-handed individuals.

The reasons for left cerebral dominance are rather obscure. O'Connor explains left-sided dominance on the basis of anatomical variance as well as on a difference in blood supply to the two hemispheres. First, the left cerebral hemisphere is larger than the right. Its inner face at the great longitudinal fissure comes very close to the midline. The corresponding inner edge of the right hemisphere is well to the right of the median line.

Second, he believes there is a distinct advantage to the left cerebral hemisphere in having a better blood supply because of the straighter course taken by the left-sided channels in reaching the cortex. The left common carotid artery ascends from the aortic arch as if it were a straight, direct prolongation of the ascending aorta. On the other hand, the right common carotid begins at the bifurcation of the innominate artery (see Figure 18). Like-

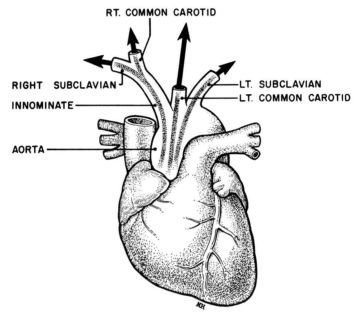

Figure 18. View of the heart and arch of the aorta, showing its three branches. Note that the left common carotid artery is a direct branch of the aortic arch, while the right common carotid artery arises from the innominate artery. (Illustration by N. Hardy.)

wise, the left vertebral artery arises from the apex of the curve in the left subclavian artery. The right vertebral artery, however, is given off by the right subclavian after the latter has described its arch and has become horizontal.

It has been claimed that this theory is invalidated by the fact that the circle of Willis (see Figure 19) provides for an equalization of the blood supply in both hemispheres. Experiments dem-

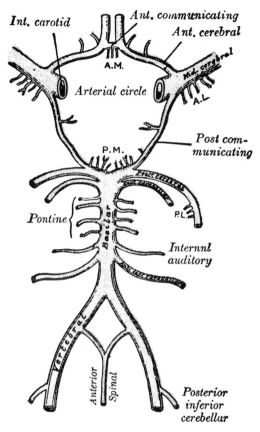

Figure 19. Diagram of the arterial circulation at the base of the brain demonstrating the circle of Willis. From Henry Gray's *Anatomy of the Human Body*, 27th Ed., edited by Charles Mayo Goss, 1959. Courtesy of Lea & Febiger, Philadelphia, Pennsylvania.

onstrate, however, that blood carried by each of the major tributaries to the Circle does not mix, but is distributed to a sharply demarcated area of the brain. According to Schmidt, the distribution of radio-opaque material injected into one internal carotid artery is strictly homolateral.

As was mentioned earlier, a distinctive feature in speech function is the dominance of one cerebral hemisphere over the other. This phenomenon is related to handedness since in right-handed individuals the left cerebral hemisphere is dominant. Evidence for this is that right hemiplegia is frequently accompanied by a language disorder. This is not usually true for left hemiplegia.

The infant uses both hands randomly. As the child grows older, there is a simultaneous development of: higher mental functions, cerebral dominance, handedness, and language function. It would appear that these functions are all interrelated. Orton (3) emphasizes the importance of cerebral dominance in relation to laterality and language function. Karlin (4) shows that a positive correlation exists between the degree of brain development, language development, and the establishment of handedness. In a group of mentally defective children, those having the highest intelligence quotients were found to have better language ability and a greater percentage of established handedness.

REFERENCES

(1) Nielsen, J. M.: *Agnosia, Apraxia, Aphasia.* New York, Paul B. Hoeber, 1946.
(2) Head, H.: *Aphasia and Kindred Disorders of Speech.* London, Cambridge University Press, 1926.
(3) Orton, S. T.: *Reading, Writing, and Speech Problems in Children.* New York, W. W. Norton & Co., 1937.
(4) Karlin, I. W., and Strazzulla, M.: Speech and Language Problems of Mentally Deficient Children. *J. Speech & Hearing Disorders,* 17:286, 1952.

Chapter 6

SENSORY ORGANS
CONCERNED WITH SPEECH

A. MECHANISM OF HEARING FOR THE
RECEPTION OF SOUND

Since it has been said that hearing is a translation of sound impulses into meaningful tones, it is important to understand the mechanism that receives the sound impulses and sends them to the brain for translation into speech and language. In most higher animals, the auditory nerve serves two mechanisms: one, the ear proper for hearing and two, a mechanism for maintaining equilibrium.

Anatomy of the Ear

The organ of hearing consists of three parts: the *external,* the *middle,* and the *inner ear.* It can also be divided into a portion for sound conduction and a part for sound reception. The conducting apparatus includes the structures found in the external and middle ear, while the receiving apparatus comprises the inner ear, especially the part known as the *cochlea.* The auditory nerve and the cortical centers for hearing are located in the temporal lobe of the cerebral hemisphere of the brain.

External Ear

The external ear is composed of the *auricle* or *pinna* and the *external acoustic meatus,* the passageway leading to the *tympanic membrane* or ear drum (see Figure 20). The auricle is movable in most animals and is of assistance in gathering sound waves. In man, the auricle has lost its mobility and can be regarded as the expanded portion of a funnel which terminates in the tympanic membrane.

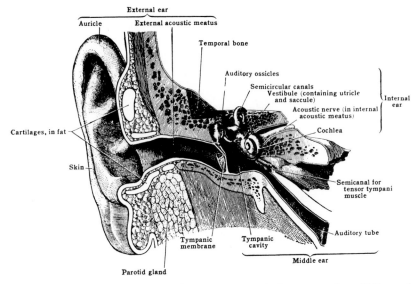

Figure 20. Diagram showing the structures of the external, middle and internal ear. From Henry Morris' *Human Anatomy*, 11th Ed., edited by J. Parsons Schaeffer, 1953. Courtesy of Blakiston Div., McGraw-Hill Book Company, Inc., New York, New York.

Middle Ear

The tympanic membrane, located at the termination of the external acoustic meatus, leads into the middle ear or *tympanic cavity* (Fig. 21). This part of the ear lies within the *temporal bone*. The outer wall of the cavity is largely formed by the flexible tympanic membrane. The inner wall, separating the middle from the inner ear, is composed of bone except for the *oval* and *round windows*. The oval window contains the footplate of the stapes. The round window, situated below the oval window, is closed by a delicate membrane. In the middle ear, three small bones called the auditory ossicles are joined together and stretch across the cavity from the tympanic membrane to the oval window. These bones are named from their shapes, the *malleus* (hammer), the *incus* (anvil), and the *stapes* (stirrup) (see Figures 20, 21).

The *eustachian tube* is the channel through which the middle ear communicates with the nasopharynx. Its chief purpose is to

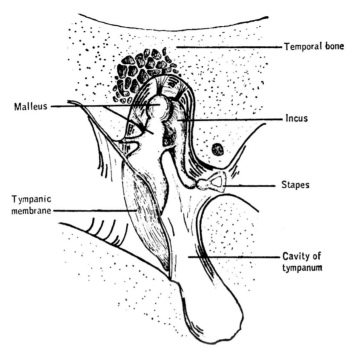

Figure 21. Diagram showing the ossicular chain of the middle ear. From Harold M. Kaplan's *Anatomy and Physiology of Speech*. Copyright 1960. Courtesy of the McGraw-Hill Book Company, Inc., New York, New York. Used by permission.

maintain equal pressure on each side of the tympanic membrane in the external and middle ear. The equalization of pressure is brought about by intermittent opening of the tube during the act of swallowing.

The tympanic cavity contains two muscles, the *tensor tympani* and the *stapedius*. Their function is to increase the tension of the tympanic membrane and the fluid within the internal ear.

The tympanic membrane transmits sound waves from the external environment to the malleus, the first member of the *ossicular chain*. The chain of bones acts as a system of levers in converting the vibrations imparted by the sound waves impinging on the tympanic membrane into stimuli of sufficient force to produce movement in the fluid of the inner ear. The energy caused by the sound vibrations is utilized by the ossicular chain to convey these vibrations to the inner ear.

Inner Ear

The inner ear or *labyrinth* is the most important part of the organ of hearing. It consists of two parts: the *osseous labyrinth,* a series of cavities within the petrous portion of the temporal bone, and the *membranous labyrinth,* a series of communicating membranous sacs and ducts within the bony cavities.

Osseous Labyrinth. The *osseous labyrinth* consists of three parts: the *vestibule, semicircular canals,* and *cochlea* (see Figure 22). These cavities contain fluid, the *perilymph,* in which the membranous labyrinth is situated.

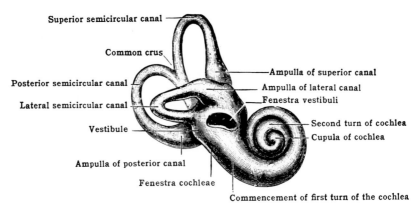

Superior semicircular canal

Common crus

Posterior semicircular canal

Lateral semicircular canal

Vestibule

Ampulla of posterior canal

Fenestra cochleae

Ampulla of superior canal

Ampulla of lateral canal

Fenestra vestibuli

Second turn of cochlea

Cupula of cochlea

Commencement of first turn of the cochlea

Figure 22. The right osseous labyrinth, in anterolateral view. Modified after Soemmering, in Henry Morris' *Human Anatomy,* 11th Ed., edited by J. Parsons Schaeffer, 1953. Courtesy of Blakiston Div., McGraw-Hill Book Company, Inc., New York, New York.

The vestibule is a passageway connecting the middle ear with the inner ear by way of the oval window. It forms the central part of the bony labyrinth from which the semicircular canals and the cochlea extend.

The bony semicircular canals are three in number: superior, posterior, and lateral. Each presents a dilatation at one end called the *ampulla.* They open into the vestibule by five orifices.

The *cochlea* forms the anterior part of the labyrinth. It contains the auditory sense organs. Its base is perforated by many apertures for the passage of the cochlear division of the *acoustic nerve.* The cochlea consists of a central axis called the *modiolus,* of a *canal,* and of the *osseous spiral lamina* which projects from the modiolus and divides the canal into two passageways called *scalae.* The upper is called the *scala vestibuli* while the lower is termed the *scala tympani.* The perilymph in the scala vestibuli connects with the perilymph that bathes the inner aspect of the oval window. This perilymph receives vibrations from the tympanic membrane by way of the ossicular chain of the middle ear. The basilar membrane stretches from the free border of the spiral lamina to the outer wall of the bony cochlea.

Membranous Labyrinth. The *membranous labyrinth* is lodged within the bony cavities and has the same general configuration as the osseous labyrinth. However, it is separated from the bony portions by the *perilymph.* The membranous labyrinth contains fluid, the *endolymph,* and on its walls the ramifications of the *acoustic nerve* are distributed. The membranous labyrinth contains two membranous sacs, the *utricle* and the *saccule* (see Figure 23). The *ductus cochlearis* is a spiral tube within the bony canal of the cochlea. One end is connected to the saccule. The dilated *ampulla* on each membranous *semicircular duct* contains a crest of neuro-epithelial cells which set up nerve impulses in response to sudden movement.

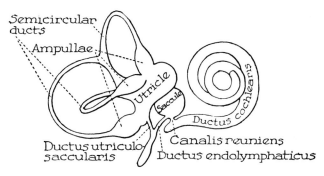

Figure 23. The membranous labyrinth. From Philip Thorek's *Anatomy in Surgery,* 2nd Ed., 1962. Courtesy of the J. B. Lippincott Company, Philadelphia, Pennsylvania.

Nerve Elements. The spiral *organ of Corti* is composed of epithelial structures placed upon the basilar membrane. The fibers of the cochlear branch of the *acoustic nerve* arise in the nerve cells of the *spiral ganglion* which is situated within the cochlea. Each cell is bipolar and sends one fiber toward the brain in the acoustic nerve, and one fiber to end in the terminal arborization around the sensory *hair cells* of the organ of Corti. The hair cells are affected by sound waves. They generate nerve impulses in the fibers of the acoustic nerve and travel by way of the *lateral lemniscus,* to end in the temporal lobe of the cerebral cortex. Two important speech centers are located in the cortex: the *transverse gyrus of Heschl and Wernicke's area.*

Physiological Considerations

Airborne sounds set up vibrations of the tympanic membrane which are transmitted to the ossicular chain of the middle ear. Vibrations are transmitted by the stapes through the oval window to the perilympth of the scala vestibuli and then to the scala tympani. From there, vibrations pass to the round window which "gives" sufficiently to permit the mechanism to operate since the fluid is not compressible. The force that drives the stapes inward is a positive sound wave. This is followed by a negative wave in which the elastic membrane of the round window contracts and reverses the fluid pressure, thus bringing the stapes back to its previous position. At the meeting point in the perilymph of a positive and negative wave, pressure is placed on the basilar membrane which stimulates the hair cells. This in turn converts the vibratory stimulus into a nerve impulse. The nerve impulse is then translated into sound in the auditory center located in the temporal lobe of the brain.

This mechanism allows the vibrations set up by the sound waves that strike the ear drum to be transmitted through the hollow cochlear duct along its full length. The end organ of hearing is the organ of Corti, consisting of nerve fibers lying along the entire floor of the cochlear duct. It is in the organ of Corti that the nerve impulses responsible for hearing originate.

The specialized cells of the organ of Corti are the internal and external rod cells and the hair cells which lie on the rod cells.

The hair cells are the essential auditory sensory elements. The sound waves conducted to the organ of Corti by the endolymph of the cochlear duct from the perilympth of the scala vestibuli affect the hair cells in some unknown way. The organ of Corti is a selective apparatus for the perception of musical sounds. It has been shown that the organ of Corti at the basal end of the cochlea makes it possible to hear high notes, while the portion at the apical end is indispensable to the hearing of low notes. Destruction of a certain portion of the cochlea is associated with inability to perceive a corresponding range of frequencies. For example, children who have hearing impairment following scarlet fever or measles develop certain so-called "tone islands." They appear to hear only restricted portions of the normal range.

Thus, the inner ear possesses a dual mechanism for hearing: the non-nervous aural microphonics and the action potential of the acoustic nerve. Sound vibrations elicit characteristic responses from each of the two mechanisms. The cochlea, acting as an electro-mechanical converter, changes mechanical vibrations into electrical potentials.

Routes of Sound Conduction

Sound waves can reach the organ of Corti by three pathways. These routes consist of the *physiological* or *ossicular route, bone conduction,* and the pathological *air route* of conduction.

1. Physiological or Ossicular Route

Sound waves conveyed to the ear are collected by the auricle, concentrated in the external auditory canal, and impinged on the tympanic membrane. Transmission is performed by the ossicular chain through the oval window to the endolymph of the membranous labyrinth where the basilar membrane of the cochlea is activated. The essential feature in this method is transmission across the middle ear via the malleus, incus, and stapes (ossicular chain). The ossicular route is the normal mechanism for hearing used by an intact ear.

2. Bone Conduction

Bone conduction forms the osseous route by which sound is transmitted to the inner ear. The ossicular chain does not play a part in this method of sound conduction. Instead, sound waves are transmitted through the outer bones of the skull to the inner ear. The middle ear is therefore by-passed. Unlike the ossicular mechanism, bone conduction plays a minor part in normal hearing because of the loss of energy in the passage of sound waves from air to the bones of the head. The mechanism of bone conduction appears to involve tiny oscillations of the skull bones which subject the fluid content of the cochlea to alternate pressures.

3. Air Route of Conduction

The air route of conduction is a *pathologic method* for the transmission of sound to the inner ear. In this method of sound conduction, sound waves usually enter the air of the middle ear directly through a hole in the tympanic membrane. This occurs when there is a perforation of the membrane or when the ossicular chain is not functioning. Sound waves then enter the inner ear through the oval window. This route is not as efficient as the physiological ossicular route. The hearing loss when sound waves are transmitted by this mechanism amounts to sixty-five decibels. Limitation of hearing to either bone conduction or air conduction results in considerable loss for the listener.

The complicated mechanism of hearing may be impaired somewhere along the line for various reasons. The question of hearing loss and its influence on speech will be considered in a later chapter.

B. ANATOMY OF THE EYE

Much of our listening is visual. For example, a child is aided in learning to speak by watching the articulators of the speaker. In addition, he learns to understand speech by looking at gestures and facial expression. Furthermore, vision is even more important when one considers the various reading disabilities found in the pre-school and school child.

The mature human eye is almost spherical, measuring 24 mm. in both horizontal and antero-posterior directions and slightly less in the vertical diameter (see Figure 24). The midpoint of the anterior curvature of the *cornea* is termed the *anterior pole* and the corresponding point on the posterior surface of the *sclera* is called the *posterior pole*. The equator of the eye is an imaginary line on the circumference of the sclera midway between the two poles. The *optic nerve* enters the eye slightly to the nasal side of the posterior pole.

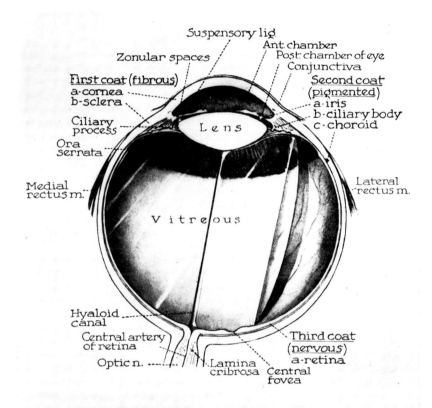

Figure 24. Horizontal section of the right eye. The eyeball has three coats (fibrous, vascular, and nervous) and three refractive media (aqueous humor, vitreous humor, and lens). From Philip Thorek's *Anatomy in Surgery*, 2nd Ed., 1962. Courtesy of the J. B. Lippincott Company, Philadelphia, Pennsylvania.

Tenon's capsule or the *fascia bulbi* is a thin fibrous membrane that surrounds the globe from the entrance of the optic nerve to a point about 3 mms. from the cornea, where it blends with the *conjunctiva.* Tenon's capsule is pierced in the region of the equator by the six *extraocular muscles* and is blended with the sheaths of these muscles. *Fascial sheaths (check ligaments)* pass from the muscle sheaths to the orbital walls and act to restrain excessive muscular movement.

The outer coat of the eyeball is covered posteriorly by the *conjunctiva,* a delicate mucous membrane. The conjunctiva is reflected onto the inner surface of the eyelids. The *lacrimal gland,* located under the supero-temporal orbital wall, secretes fluid for the lubrication of the eye. In addition, the eyelids contain the *glands of Zeis and Moll* together with the *meibomian glands,* which are responsible for secretions that keep the eye moist.

The eye consists of three concentric coats or layers (see Figure 24). The *outer* or *fibrous tunic* consists anteriorly of the *cornea* and posteriorly of the *sclera.* The *middle,* highly *vascular layer* is composed of the *iris, ciliary body,* and *choroid.* The *innermost* layer is the *nervous layer* and is called the *retina.* In addition to these coats, the eye contains various media having different refractive indices. The media consist of the *cornea, aqueous humor* (located in the *anterior chamber*), *lens,* and *vitreous body* (located in the *vitreous cavity*). Clarity of these media is essential for the proper recognition of objects in the visual field. Any obstruction of the media such as a central corneal opacity or cataractous lens change, results in loss of visual acuity.

The visual field in each eye is divided into an outer or *temporal* and an inner or *nasal* field. Rays of light from the temporal half of the visual field fall upon the nasal half of the retina, while those rays from the nasal field fall upon the temporal retina (see Figure 25). Although an image is formed upon each retina, the two are fused in consciousness into a single impression giving *binocular vision.* The *optic nerve* is formed by fibers located in the retina. Those fibers in the optic nerve arising from the nasal halves of the retinas cross in what is known as the *optic chiasm,* while the temporal fibers remain uncrossed. As a result of the crossing, each *occipital lobe* receives stimulation from the nasal half of the opposite retina and from the temporal half of the retina of the same side. Loss of vision in one half of each eye is called *hemianopia.* When the resulting blindness affects the right or the left halves of both retinas, the hemianopia is said to be *homonymous.*

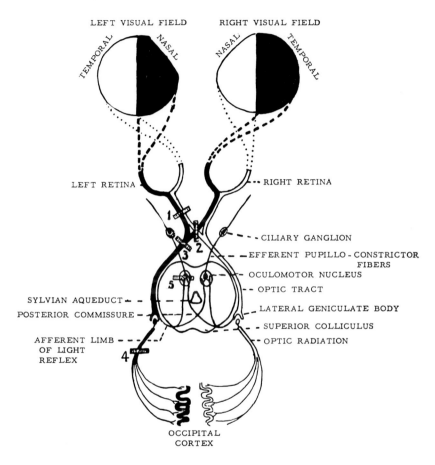

I.-OPTIC NERVE   2.-OPTIC CHIASM

Figure 25. Diagram of the eye showing its neurological structure and central connections. From Charles Best and Norman Taylor's *The Physiological Basis of Medical Practice,* 7th Ed., 1961. Courtesy of The Williams & Wilkins Company, Baltimore, Maryland.

The *optic tract* is the term used for the visual pathway between the optic chiasm and the *primary optic center,* located in the *lateral geniculate body.* After a synapse in the lateral geniculate body, visual fibers are incorporated into what is termed the *optic radiation,* which terminates in the *area striata (Brodman's area 17)* of the *occipital cortex.* Interruption of retinal impulses at various levels from the retina to the occipital cortex results in characteristic field defects as well as varying pupillary reactions. A discussion of the effects upon vision is beyond the scope of this book.

Part III

DISORDERS OF SPEECH AND LANGUAGE

Chapter 7

STUTTERING

Stuttering is of special interest to physicians, educators, psychologists, and parents since it has its onset during early childhood and manifests itself during the formative years of adolescent growth. Stuttering has been known as a speech defect since ancient times. Moses is said to have been a stutterer. In spite of stuttering having been known since the days of antiquity, there are only a few basic facts discovered about this disorder. Stuttering is not limited to, nor is it more common in, certain levels of society. It affects rich and poor, great and small, the statesman, the professional man, the scientist, and the laborer. According to Karlin (1), it occurs in about one to two per cent of the population. It is more common in boys than in girls, the ratio being approximately four to one. Its tendency to persist is more common in boys. The condition almost always begins in early childhood and, oddly enough, occurs during the years when the child's articulation as a whole tends to improve and become more distinct.

Stuttering may be defined as a disturbance in the rhythm of speech, characterized by intermittent or irregular spasmodic blocking or repetition of sounds and words. The spasm may be tonic, the muscles concerned with speech, such as those of the tongue, lips, jaw, and larynx, remaining tense and showing only a slight quiver until the sound is forced out. At other times, the spasm may be clonic, producing explosive repetition of the same sound.

ETIOLOGY

There is no definite knowledge of the cause of stuttering. There are several theories that have valid reasoning, although no theory can completely account for all the manifestations of stuttering. The interest in the study of speech and speech disorders and the progress made in this field, are mainly due to the physician, educator, and psychologist. A theory of stuttering propounded by the physician may appear to be greatly different from a theory expounded by the educator. A closer analysis, however, will reveal that perhaps the difference is mainly that of emphasis and that there is a common denominator among the various points of view. One has to be eclectic in his approach to this problem.

The earlier theories regarded stuttering as due to some abnormality of the peripheral organs of speech, such as the mouth, throat, or tongue. No one today accepts or considers these theories. To direct the stutterer's attention to his throat or mouth may only accentuate his preoccupation with the visible external structures and fix in his mind the idea that they are the seat of his problem.

Many theories have been promulgated concerning the etiology and pathogenesis of stuttering. These consist of both functional and organic hypotheses. Karlin (2) introduced a psychosomatic theory as the basis for stuttering.

Functional Theories

Many functional theories state that stuttering is a psychoneurosis, a personality disorder of social maladjustment. Coriat (3) regards stuttering as an oral neurosis in which the libido becomes fixed at the oral erotic stage of development. Appelt (4) regards stuttering as an anxiety neurosis. Greene (5) looks at stuttering as a lack of integration of the personality. Fletcher (6) views stuttering as an inability to adjust socially. In brief, stuttering, according to these theories, is an outward expression of an underlying emotional maladjustment. The outstanding emotional characteristics are fear, anxiety, and asocial behavior.

In refutation of these theories, one may say that any type of abnormality, such as stuttering, may cause the emergence of certain compensatory mechanisms which will color, to a greater or lesser extent, the daily activities of an otherwise normal person. One may well assume that the emotional characteristics of the stutterer, instead of being the cause of his stuttering, are actually the result of his poor adjustment to a difficulty which has great social implications.

Another functional group of theories has been elaborated by psychologists and educators. McDowell (7) assumes stuttering to be a habit. Johnson (8) states that stuttering is a behavior that is learned. He elaborates on this theory, and he refers to stuttering as a *diagnosogenic* and a *semantogenic* disorder. According to this theory, it is the parents' diagnosis and their attitude toward the child's speech that are the principal factors in the cause of the disorder. Johnson identifies the early repetitions of the child stutterer with the repetitions that many normal children have. It is when the parents diagnose the repetitions as stuttering, are concerned about them and begin to correct and advise the child, that stuttering results. According to this theory, stuttering is due to a faulty diagnosis in a semantic environment. While the theory that stuttering is a psychoneurosis places the emphasis on the child, the diagnosogenic theory shifts the emphasis to the parent.

It would appear from this theory that there is no such entity as stuttering until the parents make the faulty diagnosis and begin to be concerned about the child's hesitations and repetitions. It is well to remember that the majority of mothers do not make a diagnosis, and they begin to be concerned about the child's speech only when it appears to be different from the average speech of a child at the same age level. The difference, for a time, may only be in degree but not in kind. Usually, by the time the parents diagnose and begin to be concerned about the child's speech, he has already been stuttering. It is a fact that one to two per cent of the population are stutterers. Is it that the parents of this one to two per cent of children are so different from the parents of the ninety-nine per cent who do not start stuttering? How does this theory explain that there are four to five boy stutterers to every girl stutterer? This theory is simple and plausible, but does it really explain such a deep-seated disorder as stuttering? According to Brown (9), who accepts this theory, failure in the treatment of stuttering almost always occurs when the parents are unwilling or unable to accept the explanation given them by the therapist. No one can minimize the importance of parental attitudes in the treatment of stuttering. At the present stage of our knowledge, however, the clinician must assume some, if not the major, share of responsibility for failure to achieve results.

Organic Theories

The second approach to the etiology of stuttering is elaborated in the theory that stuttering is basically an organic disorder of language function. Orton (10) and Travis (11) have advanced the theory of cerebral dominance. Stuttering is considered mainly to be the result of a conflict between the two cerebral hemispheres, caused by either the lack of development of a dominant gradient or a disturbance of dominance resulting from training of the nondominant hand. Stuttering, according to this theory, is related to left-handedness in that normally left-handed children who are forced to use their right hand may stutter because of the lack of development of the dominant hemisphere.

Karlin (2) introduced a *psychosomatic theory* of stuttering in which the disorder is believed to be due to a combination of organic and psychological factors occurring approximately at the same time.

THE PSYCHOSOMATIC THEORY OF STUTTERING

In 1947, Karlin introduced his *psychosomatic theory of stuttering*. In order to understand the psychosomatic theory of stuttering, one must appreciate that most of the nerve fibers of the central nervous system and a high percentage of those in the peripheral nervous system are invested with myelin sheaths (see Figure 26). The chief constitutents of myelin are cholesterol, cerebrosides, phospholipids, and fatty acids. The myelin sheath is regarded as having an insulating function and it may also have a nutritive value to the enclosed axon.

Myelinization is regarded as correlated with function. A nerve fiber that has not been completely myelinated may transmit impulses, but the resulting action will lack precision and fine coordination. Conduction is also slower along amyelinated nerve fibers. Tilney and Casamajor (12) conclude that the deposition of myelin is coincident with the establishment of function. Keene and Hewer (13) state that even nine months after birth, myelinization of the pyramidal tracts is incomplete.

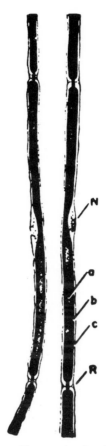

Figure 26. Medullated nerve fiber stained with osmic acid (Schafer, in Quain's Anatomy).

  a—axone
  b—myelin or medullary sheath
  c—neurolemma or sheath of Schwann (encloses the myelin sheath)
  R—node of Ranvier
  N—nucleus of the neurolemma

From Isaac W. Karlin's A Psychosomatic Theory of Stuttering, *Journal of Speech Disorders, 12*:319, 1947. Courtesy of American Speech and Hearing Association, Washington, D. C.

Observations indicate that fibers of the olivospinal tract are not even beginning to myelinate at the time of birth. It is only at the age of about eight months that these fibers begin to myelinate, at a time when the infant learns to maintain his equilibrium and to perform such coordinated movements as crawling or standing. Kuntz (14) states that the most precise and most coordinated reactions of infants are those which involve mainly conduction pathways which become myelinated early. In the spinal cord, myelinization begins in the cervical region and progresses downward. In the brain, myelinization begins in the medulla and progresses upward.

Flechsig (15) studied the development of the central nervous system in the embryonic state and in the newborn child. He originated the view that the degree of myelinization of the fibers in the central nervous system is an index of their functional capacity. He found that myelinization proceeds in the following

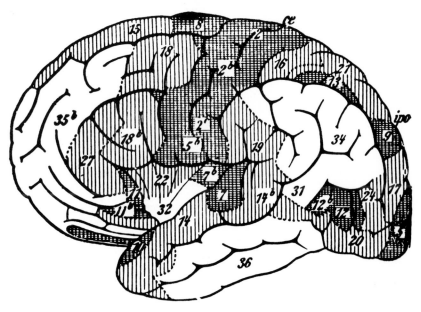

Figure 27. Lateral view of the human cerebral hemisphere, showing the cortical areas as outlined by Flechsig on the basis of differences in the time of myelinization of their nerve fibers. The primary areas (first to become myelinated) are cross-hatched; the intermediate are indicated by vertical lines; the late areas are unshaded. (Lewandowsky.) From Isaac W. Karlin's Stuttering—Evaluation and Treatment, *New York State Journal of Medicine,* 56:3719, 1956. Courtesy of the Medical Society of the State of New York, New York, N. Y.

order: first, sensory fibers; second, motor fibers; third, association fibers.

Figure 27 illustrates the order of myelinization of the various cortical areas in the brain. The first areas to be myelinated are indicated by numbers 1 to 10. The second, and later myelinization, occurs in areas 11 to 31. The last areas to undergo myelinization are shown in the areas 32 to 36. Myelinization does not proceed at a uniform rate. There are periods of acceleration and periods of decreased velocity. Myelinization may not be complete until the twentieth year of life. Flechsig (15) also makes the interesting observation that myelinization occurs earlier in the female than in the male. A comparison of Figures 27 and 28 reveals that myelinization of the speech areas is a comparatively late process in cortical development.

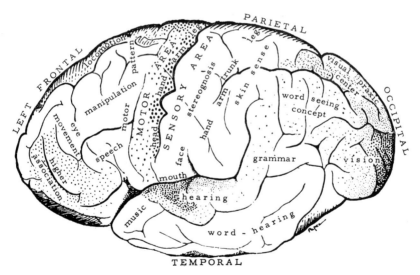

Figure 28. Lateral view of the left cerebral hemisphere, showing functional localization. From James W. Papez's *Comparative Neurology,* 1929. Courtesy of Thos. Y. Crowell Company, New York, New York.

A normally developed cortex is essential for speech. Nielsen (16) states that in its totality, symbolic thinking and expression are functions of the entire cerebral cortex. It is well established, however, that certain areas in the brain perform certain functions better than the surrounding portions of the cortex.

The average age of onset of speech is nineteen months for boys and eighteen months for girls. The observation has also been made that the child born prematurely does not differ in this respect from the normal child. McCarthy (17) states that children's speech becomes increasingly comprehensible with increase in chronological age. She also points out that speech is almost entirely comprehensible by the age of three or three and one-half years and that this development occurs earlier in girls than in boys. In the personality development of the child, it is well established that children go through a period of resistance or negativism during the third or fourth year of life.

Karlin's (2) psychosomatic theory maintains that stuttering is due to a *combination* of *organic* and *psychological* factors. The primary basic factor is a delay in the myelinization of the speech areas in the cortex. The secondary factor becomes operable when a child of three or four years of age, having a delay in myelinization, is exposed to undue emotional stress and strain during the negativistic period. This emotional stress will act like a catalytic agent in bringing forth stuttering. If judiciously managed, and if emotional stress is lessened, his speech will improve, while time is allowed for myelinization to develop so that ability to perform the fine, coordinated movements necessary for speech is fully established.

If stuttering continues, emotional factors and habit formation begin to play a greater and greater role in perpetuating stuttering. In the older child and in the adult, the emotional factors and the established neuromuscular habits become the predominating causative agents of stuttering.

At present, there is no actual anatomic proof that stuttering is basically due to a delay in myelinization of the cortical areas of the brain concerned with speech. It is a theory that requires further study and investigation. Perhaps the neuropathologists should be stimulated to take greater interest in the study of myelinization of the speech areas in individuals who were stutterers during their lifetime or had other serious speech disorders such as word deafness.

The psychosomatic theory is offered as an explanation of the fact that stuttering occurs more often in boys than in girls. First, since myelinization occurs earlier in girls, by the time the girl is three to four years old, myelinization of the speech areas in the brain is apt to be more advanced than in that of the boy. Second, the fact that myelinization may not be complete until twenty years of age, may explain why some stutterers outgrow their difficulty as they grow older and more mature. That stuttering is basically an organic disorder is supported by the fact that it has a familial tendency. Davenport (18) in discussing nervous diseases which have a genetic basis, states that stuttering has been shown by Bryant, Estabrook, and others to recur in strikingly high incidence in particular families.

DEVELOPMENT OF SYMPTOMS

Various age groups of stutterers have been investigated. The extremely small incidence of stuttering which begins in adult life, has either a purely hysterical or a definitely organic basis. The usual type of stuttering to be described is pre-eminently a disorder of early childhood. In the interest of convenience and clarity, Karlin (19) has divided the clinical history of stuttering into four groups: *preschool child, school child, adolescent and young adult,* and *adult.*

1. Onset in Preschool Child

The onset of stuttering in the preschool child is at age three to five years. Symptoms include simple repetition, hesitation, mild tension of the mouth and lips, and mild anxiety.

The onset is during the period of speech development when the child ceases to use predominantly one-word sentences and begins to express his thoughts and desires in simple sentences and later in more complex word structure. Oddly enough, stuttering begins during those years when the child's articulation as a whole tends to improve and become more distinct. The child of three or four years may begin to repeat words or sounds. He may show only an occasional slight hesitation in his speech and, while speaking, may stop suddenly as if groping for a word. A great deal has been said in recent literature to show that the early repetitions of the stutterer are in no way different from the repetitions often heard in nonstuttering children of the same age group. This is true, but the same is true of headache as a symptom, which may be due to temper tantrums or may indicate the beginning of a brain tumor. In many cases, a period of observation may be required before a definite diagnosis is made.

The normal or physiological period of hesitancy or repetition of words is of relatively short duration but will last longer in a child who is a stutterer. Van Riper (20) points out that the nonstuttering child repeats words and phrases while the young stutterer's speech has a much greater proportion of syllable repetitions. The normal child will say, "Mother, Mother, may I have, may I have . . .?" The young stutterer will say, "Muh-muh-mother, may I-I-I have . . .?" Within a few weeks or months, as the child's vocabulary increases, a certain amount of tenseness will become apparent in his repetition of words or sounds. This is due to the spasmodic contractions of the muscles concerned with speech such as those of the lips, tongue, jaw, or larynx. The spasm may be tonic, the parts involved remaining tense or showing only a slight quiver until the sound is forced through. In other cases, the spasm is clonic, producing explosive repetition of the same sounds. The child now becomes conscious of his speech difficulty. As a result, the cardinal psychological symptom of anxiety begins to appear. The family physician, or more likely the pediatrician, is the one who sees the child at this stage of stuttering.

2. School Child

In the age group of five to twelve years, the following symptoms become accentuated: tonic and clonic spasms of the mouth and lips, laryngeal spasms, muscular tensions, more pronounced anxiety, and personality maladjustments.

During this period, the symptoms of stuttering become well established. The child develops a growing awareness of his speech difficulties. Speech becomes a conscious function and is identified with the fear of stuttering. The young child may put his hand to his mouth when he begins to stutter, or he may turn his head away from the person to whom he is talking. At school, he may hold himself back from asking questions. To save him embarrassment, the teacher calls on him less frequently.

Outside of his immediate speech situations, the average child at this period of life has many absorbing interests and activities. Phantasy, at this time, is an important part of his developing personality. It tends to diminish his fear of speaking. As a result, he usually reacts to his speech difficulties with less emotion. The stuttering school child does not reveal outstanding emotional or behavioristic problems different in degree or kind from those of the nonstutterer. He does not feel himself greatly handicapped.

One may call this a latent period in the emotional influence of stuttering on the personality. At this time, the educator is the one most likely to be concerned with the problem of stuttering.

3. Adolescent and Young Adult

The adolescent and young adult usually present the classic, climactic picture of severe stuttering with marked respiratory disturbances, pronounced fear and anxiety, marked personality problems, and *invisible stuttering*. Although there is great variation in the intensity of these factors, in its most advanced form, stuttering may become the dominant factor in the individual's life.

In general, it may be said that there is no consistency as to where the severe tonic and clonic spasms may occur. In the same child, spasms may one day develop upon one set of sounds and the very next day upon different sounds. There is perhaps some tendency for the stuttering to occur more frequently and more severely upon the voiced plosives such as *b*, *d*, and *g* than upon the voiceless plosives of *p*, *t*, and *k*. In the former, not only must the articulators be released, but the larynx is used as well. In the latter, only the release of the articulators is necessary since *p, t,* and *k* are voiceless. The combined use of articulators plus laryngeal occlusion may cause more spasm in the voiced plosives.

Less evident symptoms and signs of stuttering are found in an examination of the respiratory anomalies. In normal speech, the thoracic and the abdominal phases of breathing are synchronized, inspiration being somewhat deepened and expiration prolonged. Normally, speech can be produced only during expiration. In stuttering, the synchronous activity of the thoracic and of the abdominal muscles is likely to be disrupted. Muscular spasms may involve the thoracic muscles, the abdominal muscles or the diaphragm, separately or in combination. During these spasms, the stutterer frequently tries to speak on inspiration. He often aggravates his condition by making strenuous inspiratory efforts with the head thrown back and with tense muscles of the neck and chest. He gasps for breath until, apparently exhausted, he forces out the word on expiration.

The confirmed, severe stutterer may exhibit *embolophrasia* or the insertion of meaningless words into speech. This phenomenon occurs in some aphasic and schizophrenic states. The advanced stutterer may sometimes develop a type of speech consisting of "bungling" sounds and words, or he may transpose the words of a sentence. These stutterers may become expert word jugglers to the point that as far as an outsider is concerned, there may be no apparent speech difficulty. Embolophrasia is always a conscious process on the part of the stutterer.

The advanced stutterer often has words which he is confident he can say. These words are used as *starters* to initiate the flow of speech at the beginning of a sentence. They also give him time to prepare for the phrases to follow. They are usually short exclamatory or transitional words such as: *now, and, so, well, see.*

The adolescent or young adult severe stutterer may become less sociable and more of an introvert. He may acquire a tendency to shyness. Frequently, a sense of inferiority develops. Eventually, he may indulge in self-pity and may use his speech difficulty to rationalize all his shortcomings and failures. The pattern of stuttering may be so ingrained in his personality that it may become his distinctive badge. He may experience invisible stuttering. He may think of a sentence that he would like to utter, but may feel that a certain word will give him difficulty if he were to say it. Other concomitant invisible phenomena he may experience before talking are: feelings of tension in the chest and throat, flushing of the face, palpitation, and sweating of the hands. The entire body may assume a set posture as if facing danger. This is the picture of a stutterer who has carried his difficulty with him since early childhood. He represents, to a greater or lesser degree, the climactic end result of various emotional complexes which he has built up in an effort to adjust himself to a difficulty which has great social implications. At this period it is the psychiatrist who may see the unduly disturbed stutterer or the neurotic who happens to be a stutterer.

4. Adult Stutterer

In the adult, there is usually abatement of stuttering so that the disability is markedly or moderately decreased. As the individual matures both emotionally and physically, a pattern of speech develops with a minimum of stuttering. The person has learned to cope with and to live with his difficulty. He may stutter occasionally when under stress or emotional excitement, but under normal conditions, he may speak well. While the above situation generally obtains, some adult stutterers continue to stutter badly. However, some stutterers outgrow their disability completely by the time they reach adult life.

The majority of stutterers will have less difficulty while in the following situations: singing, whispering, learning a foreign language, and reading aloud in solitude. The explanation is both physical and psychological. In whispering, since there is no laryngeal factor, one of the possibilities for spasm in stuttering is eliminated. In singing, the vowels predominate and are sustained, while the consonants are not given as much emphasis. The rhythm and melody of singing, coupled with less stress on consonants, act to minimize the possibility of stuttering. In learning a foreign language, the stutterer will not be familiar with the emotional connotations of the foreign words that he is pronouncing. Thus, he is freed from the fears that the words of his own language present. Lastly, in reading aloud in solitude, the stutterer can be more emotionally at ease, since he need not worry about the effect of his poor speech on others.

LABORATORY STUDIES

Laboratory investigations on stutterers have included respiratory tests, tests on eye movements, salivary Ph, heart rate, blood pressure, urinary creatinine, and reflex studies. None has proven to be illuminating.

The biochemical approach to stuttering was suggested by the

fact that stuttering is characterized by tonic and clonic spasms. It was naturally believed that stuttering was therefore associated with latent tetany. Tetany is characterized by hyperirritability of the nervous system and is usually caused by a deficiency of calcium and vitamin D. However, calcium and vitamin D studies on stutterers fail to demonstrate abnormal blood levels. These studies appear to rule out tetany as a possible cause of stuttering. Furthermore, tetany usually occurs much earlier than stuttering and can develop at two months of age. This tendency for its earlier occurrence, makes tetany a highly unlikely cause of stuttering.

Biochemical studies have not revealed significant differences between stutterers and nonstutterers. Karlin and Sobel (21) demonstrate the blood chemistry of stutterers and nonstutterers to be within normal limits. It is of interest, however, that statistically it is found that there is a difference, perhaps significant, in potassium levels. Stutterers have a lower potassium level than normal persons. This finding may be significant in view of the belief that potassium ions may play a part in the transmission of the nerve impulse in autonomic ganglia. A dose of potassium enhances the response of ganglion cells to preganglionic stimulation and to the action of acetylcholine.

Electroencephalographic and laterality studies of stutterers and nonstutterers do not reveal conclusive results. Investigations by Rheinberger, Karlin, and Berman (22) show that comparisons of the laterality tendencies and the electroencephalographic patterns of stutterers and nonstutterers disclose an essential similarity between the two groups. It was noted, however, that in the laterality studies, there were differences sufficient to suggest that the stutterers had somewhat less unilaterality than did the nonstutterers. Also, in the electroencephalographic studies, it was noted that children with advanced stuttering or exhibiting no progress in speech development, showed a greater incidence of positive response to hyperventilation than those whose defect was less severe. It must be emphasized that similar trends were noted in children showing asocial behavior and family history of allergy.

Karlin, Youtz, and Kennedy (23) state that endocrine disorders may play a role in distorted speech. Endocrine pathology may also play a part in stuttering, although there is no evidence at present.

Various other physiological studies have been done on stutterers. These touch on only the periphery of the problem. Thus far, such studies have not revealed any real evidence as to the etiology of stuttering. At best, the findings point only to certain leads or trends that the stutterer exhibits. At present, the only outstanding group of factors which set apart stuttering from other types of speech defects are the emotional or psychological factors. It is principally around these factors that the present day treatment of stuttering has been based.

PROGNOSIS

As to prognosis, "Once a stutterer, always a stutterer" has been the opinion of some well-known authorities in this field. At the other extreme, it has been claimed that a cure is possible for all. The laity as well as many physicians rely freely on the belief that, "The child will outgrow it." The time-honored advice given by the pediatrician, who is usually the first person that the mother consults, is: "Ignore it. Every child repeats. He will outgrow it." But do they all outgrow it? Many children of three or four years of age begin to show the early signs of stuttering. The parents are concerned and talk about the condition, but in a relatively short time and with no therapy, the children go on to normal speech. Other children begin with the same mild symptoms as the previous group, but soon show definite stuttering. The parents may seek advice and, with minimal therapy or without it, the children stop stuttering within a few months. Perhaps in a year, their speech becomes normally fluent. Milisen and Johnson (24) in a study of approximately 8,000 public school children, stated that of the total number of stutterers, forty-two per cent outgrew the disorder without clinical assistance. In the authors' clinical experience, about fifty per cent outgrow stuttering. The other fifty per cent of stutterers begin to block in a similar way to the previous group. However, their stuttering continues and frequently becomes worse. This group forms the one to two per cent of the population who will continue to stutter.

Within this last group, perhaps ninety per cent of the parents take the advice of the physician or neighbor and ignore the defect. Their children become full stutterers, with all its symptoms and complexes. The remaining ten per cent of the children in the last group receive what is believed today to be competent help.

There are no tests today by which one can tell whether the child who begins to hesitate unduly or to repeat words and sentences, will start stuttering or whether he will have normal speech. Likewise, no one can possibly predict which child will recover from his stuttering. The diagnosis of stuttering can be made only when the child stutters as he talks. The rule should be that every child of three or four years of age who begins to hesitate and repeats words and sentences sufficiently to be noticed, should be treated as early as possible. The hope is to rescue some of the children who receive no therapy at all.

TREATMENT

Perhaps no other human disorder has received so many types of treatment and claims of cure as stuttering. From Demosthenes, who is said to have cured his handicap by filling his mouth with pebbles while trying to declaim louder than the roar of the ocean waves, to walking upside down to increase blood flow to the brain, various cures for stuttering have been reported by professionals, quacks, and parlor amateurs. Although there are no scientific studies and no statistical tables reporting the results of this type of treatment, each one knows of at least one person cured of stuttering.

The infant hears many sounds around him which at first are without significance. He soon learns that certain sounds or words are associated with certain experiences, and these in turn acquire an emotional tone. It must be remembered that the young child's life is richly emotional and that he does not acquire all the speech sounds simultaneously. West, Ansberry, and Carr (25) have shown that there is a definite order of progression in the development of speech sounds. Furthermore, Karlin and Kennedy (26) have indicated that the development of speech does not proceed at the same rate in every child.

Karlin (1) views the treatment of stuttering as both medical and educational. It should be medical because the physician, by his training, views the total personality of the child both from physical and mental aspects. He gains insight into the personal life of the child and into environmental factors surrounding him. Using these studies, the physician makes an effort to provide for the child the optimal conditions of health and emotional stability. Treatment must also be educational because the trained teacher of speech can help to observe and to analyze the various forms and shades of articulatory disturbance that the stutterer may present. The specialist in speech will then endeavor to understand the child's interests, to improve his attitude toward speech, and to provide him with a good speech pattern. As in all difficulties dominated by emotional factors, it is the personality of the person who treats the condition, as well as the training itself, that determines the effectiveness of the treatment.

Speech Treatment for Preschool Child

Treatment should begin as soon as stuttering is noticed. The rule should be that every child of three or four years of age who begins to hesitate and repeat sounds or syllables sufficiently to be noticed, should be treated as early as possible. The best time and the best results obtained in the treatment of stuttering are in its inception.

The basis for the treatment of stuttering of the preschool child is to allow further maturation of the cortical speech areas, so that maximum stability and neuromuscular coordination develop in the function of speech. At the same time, one must try to hold to a minimum the emotional factors which complicate and accentuate the disorder. The goal is to lessen emotional tension and thereby establish a favorable background for speech conditions at home, so that time is allowed for the normal progress of myelinization to proceed.

Examination of the preschool child begins first with an adequate history from the parents of the child's speech makeup from birth. Past medical history should include diseases and any deviation of behavior from the normal growth and development. A complete physical examination follows. Vision and hearing should be checked, and any defects corrected if possible. The parents, especially the mother, may be dominated by the feeling of guilt induced by reading or hearing some psychological concepts about stuttering. She may believe that something she did or said has produced the "emotional block" that caused the difficulty. The parents must be relieved of this sense of guilt. They should be told that the development of speech is subject to individual variations and that environmental influences will condition a child to certain types of behavior and performance. A great deal has been said about the child's need for love, security, and a feeling of belonging. Important as these factors are, the child also needs positive guidance. The parents should have a feeling of certainty in handling the child, and they should not interfere with one another in their everyday dealings with him. There should be no fear that stuttering is "contagious" or imitative.

Karlin (27) stresses that the preschool child's attention should not be drawn to his speech difficulty. Members of the family must avoid any outward emotional reactions when the child stutters. The speech environment should be the best possible. The parents should talk in the child's presence in a relaxed manner. They should observe the conditions under which the child talks best, and these situations should be encouraged. Situations that aggravate stuttering should be avoided. Undue fatigue is to be avoided since stuttering increases with fatigue. A period of relaxation should be provided every day during which time the mother should read to the child in a calm and easy manner.

The question is frequently posed about the relationship between handedness and stuttering. The consensus today is that there is no actual connection between handedness and stuttering. However, Karlin and Strazzulla (28) show that there is a relationship between cortical development, language development, and handedness. The better the unilaterality as exhibited by handedness and the more advanced the cortical development, the better the language function. A child with a speech or language disorder, and this includes the stutterer, should be encouraged to use and develop his preferential hand, be it left or right. The significant factor is the method used in the enforcement of handedness.

This is the *indirect method* of treatment of the stutterer during the preschool period. He is not to be made conscious of his defect, and no direct speech therapy is given. The treatment is mainly through the parents. To ignore the defect or to encourage the false idea that stuttering is nonexistent, and that every child hesitates when he talks, is to waste much valuable time. The keynote to the problem of stuttering in the preschool child is early recognition and indirect treatment.

Speech Therapy for School Child, Adolescent, and Young Adult

The treatment of the school child, the adolescent, and the young adult is a much more difficult problem. Since social contacts become wider and more complex as children grow older, individual problems and their adjustments have to be considered. The problem of stuttering should be discussed freely and openly in contrast to the indirect approach for the preschool child. This will remove some of the aura of mystery that surrounds stuttering. An effort should be made to lessen the stutterer's fears and anxieties and to increase his self confidence. School adjustments may have to be made. A pattern of speech must be provided by the speech clinician, physician, and educator which will be best for him. While many of these problems have to be worked out individually, group therapy has its value and should be used.

The role of the speech clinician is important at the school, adolescent, and adult levels. The teacher of speech uses the play technique in winning the child's friendship and cooperation. She demonstrates a good speech pattern not only for the child but for the parents. She reads stories and rhymes to the child and has him repeat them. She stimulates his interest and provokes spontaneous conversation and questions, striving constantly for good speech.

Karlin (29) believes high points in *direct* remedial speech work for the school child, adolescent, and young adult include:

1. *Relaxation.* The stutterer has to learn how to relax while he talks, and be able to overcome muscle tension when he has difficulty in articulating a sound.

2. *Respiration.* The stutterer must learn to coordinate breathing and talking. The common advice, "Take a deep breath," produces only greater tension and fatigue.

3. *Phrasing.* The stutterer must acquire an ability to establish pauses in his speech to control phrasing.

4. *Rate Control.* Prolongation of vowel sounds helps the stutterer overcome muscle tension and is useful as a rate control.

Ancillary Methods of Treatment

Drug therapy may be of value and should be tried. In children who show decided tensions and spasms at the onset of treatment, Karlin used for shorter periods either bromides or neostigmine and atropine. Benadryl and reserpine appear to be of definite value at times. Karlin (27) is of the opinion that phenobarbital makes the children more tense causing accentuation of stuttering. Meduna (30) advocates carbon dioxide therapy and reports good results with some stutterers.

Psychoanalysis should help the adjustment of the unduly emotionally disturbed stutterer or the psychoneurotic who happens to be a stutterer. Psychoanalysis, however, cannot be advocated as a cure for stuttering. Freud states that psychoanalysis will not cure stuttering. Brill (31) states that only a few of those stutterers who receive psychoanalytic treatment are ultimately cured in any real sense. Those he helped were neurotics who developed stuttering later on in life.

Hypnosis is not a cure for stuttering. With some cases, hypnosis may produce temporary improvement, while in others, after the temporary improvement, stuttering may be worse than before.

Summary of Treatment

Karlin and Kennedy (32) summarized their approach to therapy in stuttering, which still holds true today. The following is an outline of their methods:

I. Complete physical and neurological examination
II. Mental test to determine child's intelligence quotient
III. Interview with parents with special emphasis on:

A. Developmental history of the child
    1. Type of delivery
    2. Onset of teething
    3. Onset of sitting
    4. Onset of walking
    5. Onset of talking
    6. Muscular control; coordination
    7. Handedness

B. Environmental history
    1. Social and educational history of family
    2. Emotional history of family
    3. Number of siblings
    4. Parent-child relationship
    5. Child-sibling relationship
    6. Type of discipline in the home
    7. Sleeping arrangements

C. Personal history of child
    1. Chronological age and educational progress
    2. Illness; mother's attitude and handling
    3. Habits or neurotic traits, such as bed wetting, thumb sucking, and masturbation
    4. Temperamental and emotional attitudes such as timidity, aggression, self-reliance, friendliness, irritability, affection, coldness, and a feeling of security

D. Speech history
    1. Speech history of family
    2. Language spoken at home
    3. Onset of patient's speech including babbling
    4. Type of early speech
    5. Onset of stuttering
    6. Cause of stuttering as given by parent
    7. Type and degree of stuttering
    8. Situations in which stuttering is most pronounced, lessened, or absent
    9. Any prolonged remissions from stuttering and the apparent cause
    10. Parents' attitude toward the defect
    11. Child's attitude toward his defect
    12. Social reactions of schoolmates and playmates
    13. Method of correction attempted by family or by other agents
    14. Child's reaction to corrective methods
    15. Devices child may use to help himself

16. Overt emotional reactions accompanying the disorder, such as blushing and tics
17. Other defects of speech

IV. Interview with child
  A. To establish rapport
  B. To pave the way for further contact
  C. To analyze speech of child
  D. To gain information about:

    1. Earliest recollections
    2. Play life
    3. Fears and emotional conflicts
    4. Attitude toward family, companions, and school
    5. Attitude toward speech difficulty and toward corrective measures
    6. Interests and ambitions

V. Division of mentally normal children into the following groups:
  A. Preschool child
  B. School child, adolescent, and young adult

VI. Program of treatment for the preschool child (Group A)

  A. Interview with parents and child as outlined (I, II, III, IV)

  B. Method of treatment
    More indirect approach than with the school child
    (a) Child not made conscious of his defect
    (b) Emphasis placed on the imitation of the good speech pattern set by the speech teacher
    (c) Parents to give child a good speech pattern, which is characterized by smoothness, fluidity, and ease of initiation

  C. Intelligent cooperation of the parents stressed as an important factor in the therapy of the preschool child.

VII. Program of activities for the school child, adolescent, and young adult (Group B)

  A. Direct approach: child's attention directed to the importance of good speech

  B. Individual conferences
    1. Patient seen individually from time to time and the various factors (IV, D) gone into in greater detail in an effort to better understand child's attitude and problems
    2. Patient given to understand that the reason for these discussions is the desire to help him

3. Special emphasis placed on the emotional problems that may be present at home, in school, or outside
4. Patient given insight into and understanding of his problems, and a cooperative attempt made to solve them or resolve them
5. Attempt made to develop in child a feeling of security and self-confidence
6. Technique of relaxation given
7. Suggestive treatment applied

C. Group activities and procedures
   1. Progressive relaxation
      (a) Purposes
         (1) To lessen bodily tension
         (2) To induce control of body and of emotions
      (b) Activities
         (1) Tensing of muscles later to be relaxed
         (2) Relaxing progressively, beginning with the largest group of muscles and proceeding to the smallest
         (3) Relaxation of whole muscular arc
   2. Breath control
      (a) Purposes
         (1) To induce low, controlled, easy breathing
         (2) To lessen tension in neck and shoulders
         (3) To develop a more adequate breath span, with emphasis on controlled exhalation
         (4) To coordinate breathing and phrasing
      (b) Procedures
         (1) Discussion of relation between exhalation and inhalation in speech
         (2) Demonstration of diaphragmatic breathing

      (c) Activities
         (1) Group exercise in controlled breathing
         (2) Slow counting on controlled expiration
         (3) Increasing the breath span; counting from one to five and from one to ten, progressively, for each exhalation
         (4) Good duration pattern, giving full value to vowels instead of shortening them
         (5) Rhythmic phrases and sentences to be repeated for smoothness of phrasing with more frequent breath groups without damaging the inherent rhythm
   3. Reading
      (a) Purpose: synthesis of objectives mentioned

    (b) Procedure: group imitation of good pattern of speech, followed by individual presentation of it, through medium of rhythmic poetry and prose

    (c) Activities

        (1) Good speech pattern given by teacher through the medium of rhythmic poetry and prose

        (2) Stutterer reads the selection with the teacher, then with the group

        (3) Stutterer reads individually

        (4) Stutterer again listens to good speech pattern

        (5) Stutterer attempts to follow it alone

4. Socialized speech activities

    (a) Purpose: to place stutterers in the situation which most nearly approximates a situation met in daily life

    (b) Procedures

        (1) Games

        (2) Club activities

    (c) Activities

        (1) Language games, such as Geography and Coffee Pot

        (2) Informal dramatizations

        (3) Pantomimes

        (4) Talks by the patients

        (5) Club work: students organized into a club in which all the activities are carried out by them with a minimum amount of supervision

"Cast out the stuttering devil" has been the cry throughout the ages. Some progress has been made, but the search is still going on. There are those who say, "Once a stutterer, always a stutterer," and there are those who contend that the therapeutic goal is achieved when the stutterer stops being concerned about his defect. These are purely negative attitudes. If one is educated to make an early diagnosis of stuttering and immediately institutes a program of therapy for this disorder, one can frequently aid the child in overcoming this oftentimes disabling speech impediment.

REFERENCES

(1) Karlin, I. W.: Stuttering—the Problem Today. *J.A.M.A., 143*:732, June 24, 1950.

(2) Karlin, I. W.: A Psychosomatic Theory of Stuttering. *J. Speech Dis., 12*:319, September, 1947.

(3) Coriat, I. H.: *Stammering; a Psychoanalytic Interpretation.* Nervous and Mental Disease Monograph Series, No. 47. New York, Nervous and Mental Disease Publishing Co., 1928.

(4) Appelt, A.: *The Real Cause of Stammering and Its Permanent Cure.* London, Methuen & Co., 1911.

(5) Greene, J. S.: The Stutter-Type Personality and Stuttering. *New York J. Med.,* 36:757, May 15, 1936.

(6) Fletcher, J. M.: *The Problem of Stuttering. A Diagnosis and a Plan of Treatment.* New York, Longmans, 1928.

(7) McDowell, E. V.: Educational and Emotional Adjustments of Stuttering Children. *Contributions to Education No. 314.* New York, Teachers College, Columbia University, 1928, p. 1.

(8) Johnson, W.: *People in Quandaries; The Semantics of Personal Adjustment.* New York, Harper & Brothers, 1946.

(9) Brown, S. F.: Advising Parents of Early Stutterers. *Pediatrics,* 4:170, August, 1949.

(10) Orton, S. T.: *Reading, Writing and Speech Problems in Children: A Presentation of Certain Types of Disorders in the Development of the Language Faculty.* New York, W. W. Norton & Co., 1937.

(11) Travis, L. E.: Speech Pathology: *A Dynamic Neurological Treatment of Normal Speech and Speech Deviations.* New York, D. Appleton & Co., 1931.

(12) Tilney, F., and Casamajor, L.: Myelinogeny as Applied to the Study of Behavior. *Arch. Neurol. Psychiat.,* 12:1, July, 1924.

(13) Keene, M. F. L., and Hewer, E. E.: Some Observations on Myelination in the Human Central Nervous System. *J. Anat.,* 66:1, October, 1931.

(14) Kuntz, A.: *A Textbook of Neuro-Anatomy.* Philadelphia, Lea & Febiger, 1942.

(15) Flechsig, P.: *Meine Myelogenetische Hirnlehre Mit Biographischer Einleitung.* Berlin, Julius Springer, 1927.

(16) Nielsen, J. M.: *Agnosia, Apraxia, Aphasia.* New York, Paul B. Hoeber, Inc., 1946.

(17) McCarthy, D. A.: *The Language Development of the Preschool Child.* Institute of Child Welfare. Monograph Series No. 4. Minneapolis, University of Minnesota Press, 1930.

(18) Davenport, C. B.: Heredity and Eugenics in Relation to Medicine. *The Oxford Medicine* 1:519, 1934.

(19) Karlin, I. W.: Stuttering; Evaluation and Treatment. *New York J. Med.,* 56:3719, December 1, 1956.

(20) Van Riper, C.: *Speech Correction: Principles and Methods.* New York, Prentice-Hall, 1963.

(21) Karlin, I. W., and Sobel, A. E.: A Comparative Study of the Blood Chemistry of Stutterers and Non-stutterers, *Speech Monogr.,* 7:75, 1940.

(22) Rheinberger, M. D., Karlin, I. W., and Berman, A. B.: Electro-encephalographic and Laterality Studies of Stuttering and Non-stuttering Children. *Nerv. Child,* 2:117, 1943.

(23) Karlin, I. W., Youtz, A. C., and Kennedy, L.: Distorted Speech in Young Children. *Am. J. Dis. Child.,* 59:1203, June, 1940.

(24) Milisen, R., and Johnson, W.: A Comparative Study of Stut-terers. *Arch. Speech* 1:61, 1936.

(25) West, R., Ansberry, M., and Carr, A.: *The Rehabilitation of Speech.* New York, Harper & Brothers, 1957.

(26) Karlin, I. W., and Kennedy, L.: Delay in the Development of Speech. *Am. J. Dis. Child.,* 51:1138, May, 1936.

(27) Karlin, I. W.: Stuttering. *Arch. Pediat.,* 63:23, January, 1946.

(28) Karlin, I. W., and Strazzulla, M.: Speech and Language Prob-lems of Mentally Deficient Children. *J. Speech & Hearing Disorders,* 17:286, September, 1952.

(29) Karlin, I. W.: Stuttering. *Am. J. Nursing* 48:42, January, 1948.

(30) Meduna, L. J.: *Carbon Dioxide Therapy: A Neurophysiological Treatment of Nervous Disorders.* Springfield, Thomas, 1950.

(31) Brill, A. A.: *Basic Principles of Psychoanalysis.* Garden City, New York, Doubleday & Co., Inc., 1949.

(32) Karlin, I. W., and Kennedy, L.: Stuttering: Problem and Sug-gested Treatment. *Am. J. Dis. Child.,* 55:383, February, 1938.

Chapter 8

DISORDERS OF ARTICULATION

MANY SPEECH clinicians and pathologists, if asked to rank the relative importance of various speech defects, would place disorders of articulation first. On the other hand, some investigators are inclined to believe that articulatory difficulties are of minor importance even though many of these defects defy correction.

ARTICULATION AND INTELLIGIBILITY

Articulation of the sounds of language is basic to intelligibility of communication. There are, however, other aspects of the phonetic structure of language that are essential to intelligible speech and that are closely related to articulation. In addition to articulation of sounds of language, these other factors are: length or duration of sound; stress on syllables of words according to usage in the language; logical stress on words in groups; syllable division; logical phrasing of words into thought groups; and intonation appropriate to the language spoken and to the thought being conveyed.

Sounds of a given language must be taught systematically in order to improve articulation. Our faulty English alphabet contains twenty-six letters, but our language contains forty sounds. What are these sounds, and how are they articulated? Since one must first become familiar with the normal articulatory mechanism before one can recognize and treat the pathological defects in articulation, the authors have decided to divide this chapter into two parts. The first division will explore the normal phonetic structure of the English language while the second part will concern itself with the defects in articulation.

A. PHONETIC STRUCTURE OF THE ENGLISH LANGUAGE

The Sounds of English

The sounds of the English language have been identified and classified as to articulation by phoneticians from England, the

PRONUNCIATION KEY

Word		Merriam-Webster	International Phonetic Alphabet	Key Number
a	father	ä	ɑ:	1
	stand	ă	æ	2
	walk	ô	ɔ:	3
	last	ȧ	a	4
	alone	ă	ə	5
	name *(D)*	ā	eĭ	6
	fare *(D)*	â	εə̆	7
b	bib	b	b	8
c	s as in city; k as in car			
	church	ch	tʃ	9
d	did	d	d	10
e	met	ĕ	e	11
	meet	ē	i:	12
	here	ē̇	iə̆	13
f	fife	f	f	14
g	give	g	ɡ	15
h	hat	h	h	16
i	tin	ĭ	ı	17
	girl	û	⌣:	18
	time *(D)*	ī	aĭ	19

Figure 29. The sounds of English, using the International Phonetic Alphabet and the Merriam-Webster diacritic markings. From Louise Gurren's *Better Speech*, Living Language Series, 1957. Courtesy of Crown Publishers, Inc., New York, New York.

United States, Scotland, and other parts of the English speaking world such as Australia, New Zealand, South Africa, and Canada. Gurren's Figure 29 shows all the sounds of English, using the International Phonetic Alphabet and the Merriam-Webster diacritic markings.

Since English is spoken over such a wide area, there are differences in pronunciation in various regions. In general, however, for improved intelligibility through improved articulation, it is advisable to teach sounds that are recognized as good speech

PRONUNCIATION KEY

	Word	Merriam-Webster	International Phonetic Alphabet	Key Number
j	judge	j	dʒ	20
k*	cook	k	ᴋ	21
l	leave	l	l	22
m	main	m	m	23
n	net	n	n	24
	sing	ng	ŋ	25
o	on	ŏ	ɒ	26
	obey	ȯ	o	27
	book	ŏŏ	u	28
	home *(D)*	ō	oŭ	29
	boy *(D)*	oi	ɔĭ	30
	down *(D)*	ou	aŭ	31
	poor *(D)*	ŏŏ	ʊə̆	32
	shore	ō	ɔə̆	33
p*	pipe	p	p	34
q	kw as in quick	kw	kw	
r	real	r	ɹ	35
s	six	s	s	36
	sure	sh	ʃ	37
	measure	zh	ʒ	38
t*	tent	t	t	39
	thin	th	θ	40
	then	~~th~~	ð	41
u	blue	oo	u:	42
	up	ŭ	ʌ	43
v	velvet	v	v	44
w	wear	w	w	45
wh	where	wh	ʍ	46
x	ks as in six; ksh as in luxury; gz as in exact; gzh as in luxurious			
y	yellow	y	j	47
z	zebra	z	z	48

*p, t, ᴋ with a slight puff of breath before a vowel and before a pause; without a puff of breath before another consonant.

FIGURE 29 (cont'd.).

anywhere. In other words, by teaching that pronunciation which is free from peculiarities, the clinician is preparing the speaker for communication that will be useful wherever English is spoken.

One of the goals of the speech clinician is to raise the intelligibility of the speaker by improving his articulation. Other equally important goals include the following: first, changing the speaker's attitude toward speech; second, improving, where necessary, the use of vocabulary, structure, and language. While working on the improvement of articulation, the clinician is often able to change the speaker's attitude toward speech, giving him confidence by showing the speaker how the sounds are made. The clinician may also improve vocabulary and grammatical usage by teaching sounds in words, phrases, and sentences for practice in articulation.

It is very important for the speech clinician to be able to pronounce the sounds reasonably accurately himself. Experiments have shown that the *stimulation method* combined with the *phonetic method* is most effective. These methods combine repetition of the sound by the speech clinician with a description of the phonetic placement of the sound. The response by the child and its comparison to that of the clinician follows. If the speech clinician's speech is not clear, the patient will not be able to give a clear response.

English Vowels

Vowels have been classified according to the *part of* the *tongue* used in saying them, the *position* of that part *of* the *tongue,* the *position of* the *lips,* and the *length* or quantity of the vowel. The chart of the English vowels shown in Figure 30, provides a clear way of seeing the various aspects of the articulation of these sounds. Length is indicated on the chart by placing two dots after the letter representing the sound. The lips are rounded for all the sounds on the right side of the chart except the last one. The words *front, mid,* and *back* refer to the part of the tongue used in saying the sounds. The words *high, half high, half low,* and *low* refer to the relative position of the front, middle, or back of the tongue while voicing a given sound. The letters used are those of the International Phonetic Association.

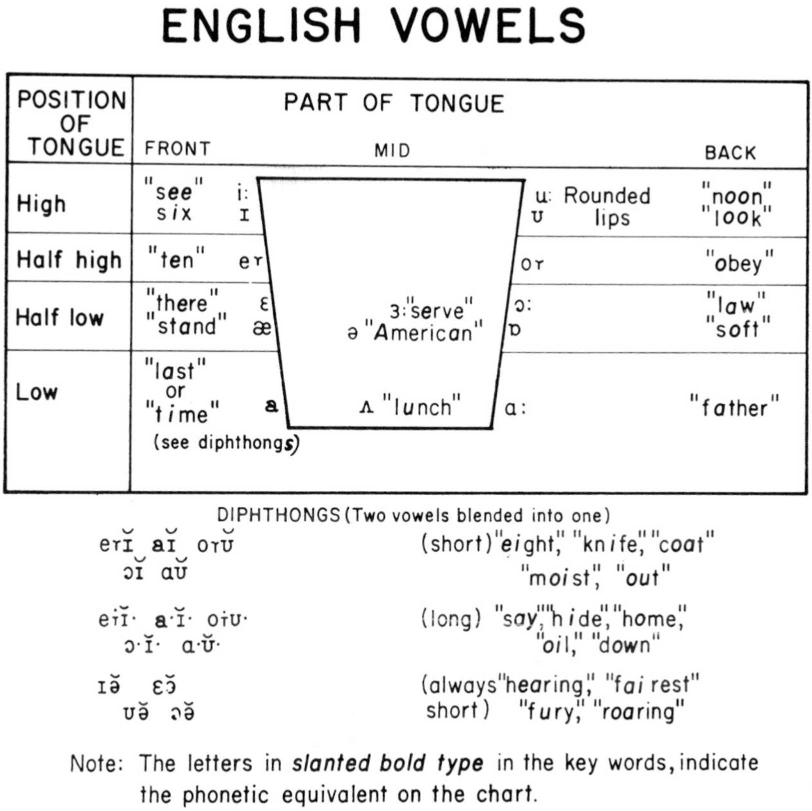

ENGLISH VOWELS

POSITION OF TONGUE	PART OF TONGUE		
	FRONT	MID	BACK
High	"see" i: s*i*x ɪ		u: Rounded "noon" ʊ lips "look"
Half high	"ten" eɤ		oɤ "obey"
Half low	"there" ε "stand" æ	3:"serve" ə "American"	ɔ: "law" ɒ "soft"
Low	"last" or "t*i*me" a (see diphthongs)	ʌ "lunch"	a: "father"

DIPHTHONGS (Two vowels blended into one)

eɤɪ̆ aɪ̆ oɤʊ̆ ɔɪ aʊ̆	(short) "*ei*ght," "kn*i*fe," "c*oa*t" "m*oi*st," "*ou*t"
eɤɪ̆· a·ɪ̆· oɤʊ̆· ɔ·ɪ̆· a·ʊ̆·	(long) "s*ay*," "h*i*de," "h*o*me," "*oi*l," "d*ow*n"
ɪə̆ εə̆ ʊə̆ ɔə̆	(always "h*ea*ring," "f*ai* rest" short) "f*u*ry," "r*oa*ring"

Note: The letters in *slanted bold type* in the key words, indicate the phonetic equivalent on the chart.

Figure 30. The English vowels and diphthongs, showing part and position of tongue for their articulation. International phonetic symbols are used (after Gurren).

One of the problems in connection with the understanding of English vowels is the fact that the alphabet contains only five letters to represent vowels: *a, e, i, o, u*. In addition, *y* is frequently pronounced as a vowel. The spoken language, however, contains fifteen vowels and nine diphthongs. The five letters of our written language cannot represent the fifteen vowels and nine diphthongs that are used in the spoken language. It is, therefore, very important for the speech clinician to differentiate between sounds and letters. Letters are symbols we write and see. Sounds are utterances we say and hear. Both are linguistic phenomena. They should not be confused with one another, especially since English spelling is so unphonetic.

English Consonants

Consonants are classified as to *point* and *manner* of articulation as contrasted to vowels which are classified in terms of part and position of tongue, lip rounding, and length. There are six points for articulation of English consonants: the lips; the upper teeth and lower lip; the teeth; the upper gum ridge; the hard palate; and the soft palate. The manner of articulation includes the following aspects: voiced or unvoiced sounds; stop sounds or fricatives; vowel-like consonants; and nasal consonants (see Table IV, page 59).

Gurren's Table IV indicates the point and manner of articulation of English consonants. The letters printed in bold face represent the voiced consonants.

It is important to note that another aspect of articulation of consonants concerns itself with length. In English, a consonant is lengthened before a pause if it follows a short vowel in a stressed syllable. In the word *ham,* the *m* follows the short vowel æ. Therefore, the *m* is lengthened. On the other hand, in the word *home,* the *m* follows the long diphthong oīŭ·. Therefore, the *m* is not long. Some of these details may seem unimportant, but articulation of sounds includes duration. Thus, appropriate duration, or quantity, heightens intelligibility.

Three factors must be provided for the normal articulation of any given consonant. First, the production of vocal tone is necessary if the sound is voiced. Second, sufficient air pressure must be built up in the mouth and in the throat. Third, the proper adjustment of the articulators must be made. The production of vocal tone is provided by the approximation of the vocal cords. The escape of air between them causes a vibration or a flutter of the edges of each vocal cord. The vocal tone is the result of this vibration. The creation of sufficient air pressure depends upon the force of the respiratory muscles to drive the column of air through the nose and mouth. The closing of the nasopharyngeal passage is accomplished by the raising of the velum and the simultaneous contraction of the superior constrictors of the pharynx, forming Passavant's cushion.

Stress on Syllables of Words

Practice in the articulation of sounds is a basic step toward the improvement of intelligibility. Single sounds, however, must be put into words and connected speech. A very important aid to increased effectiveness is appropriate stress on syllables of words.

Stress may be defined as uttering a syllable with greater force or volume than is given the others in a word of more than one syllable. Stress, or lack of it, may change the articulation of sounds in a word. Greater force, or volume, heightens the perceptibility of the syllable that is given the stress. The vowel in the stressed syllable is clearer than those in the unstressed syllables in the English language. Thus, the stressed syllable plays an important role in "carrying the message."

There are two aspects of stress to be considered: *location* and *degree*. If the location of the stress is misplaced, neither the volume nor the articulation of the sounds are those the listener expects to hear in a given word. It is unfortunate that there are no reliable rules for location of stress in English as there are in French, Spanish, and Italian. The degree of stress is equally as important as the location. In English, there are three degrees of stress: strong, secondary, and weak. The word, "association," indicates the various degrees of stress. The fourth syllable, *a*, contains the strong stress. The second syllable, *so*, contains the secondary stress. The other syllables are unstressed or weak.

It is important for the speech clinician to remember that while he is working on the improvement of the articulation of sounds, the question of stress on words of more than one syllable should be dealt with through instruction and practice.

Stress on Words in Groups

When the speech clinician applies practice of articulation to words in groups, in phrases, and in sentences, there will be some words in the group that logically receive more stress than others. These words gain heightened perceptibility because of their importance in the communication of the idea to be conveyed. This heightened volume often changes the articulation of the sounds in the words stressed.

In general, words that carry stress are the nouns, verbs, adjectives, and adverbs. The auxiliary *to have* and the verb *to be*, on the other hand, usually are spoken in the unstressed or weak form.

Strong and Weak Forms of Words

Many words have both strong, or stressed, and weak forms. Articles, prepositions, personal pronouns, the word *not*, some conjunctions, the verb *do* in some instances, and many others, have both a strong and a weak form. In the contractions *didn't*, *wouldn't*, *shouldn't*, and *couldn't*, the word *not* is weakened by converting it to *n't*. These words are difficult for children to pronounce. The use of weak forms and contractions is essential to fluent speech, since they give heightened perceptibility to the stressed words.

Syllable Division

To increase intelligibility through improvement in smoothness and fluency, it is often helpful to explain to the child the number of syllables or impulses of utterance in a word. Some children with poor articulation say *father* (fa-ther), for example, as though it were *faaaa*. After practicing the articulation of the *th*, it is helpful to work on the two beats or impulses of the word, saying *fa ther*, being sure to give length to the *a*, strong stress to the syllable *fa*, and weak stress to the syllable *ther*. Many children benefit from this kind of instruction. The speech clinician must be careful, however, to keep the pronunciation natural, to avoid all artificiality or exaggeration and to put the word together again for practice in phrases and sentences. Length, strong and weak stress and syllable division are closely bound up with what is popularly called the "rhythm of the language."

Phrasing

Phrasing is the grouping of words according to meaning. All those words that logically belong together are uttered in one breath or thought group. Uneven phrasing is one of the causes of low intelligibility in communication. Imagine, for example, a speaker, having run upstairs, trying to communicate a message when he is completely out of breath. His voice will be indistinct. His phrasing will be irregular because he has insufficient breath to say a complete thought or part of a thought in one breath group. The listener will not be able to understand him, not necessarily because of his voice, but rather because of his poor phrasing.

Childern with poor articulation have difficulty in phrasing their thoughts as they speak. Their difficulty in articulating sounds often breaks their thoughts into uneven phrases that are difficult for the listener to follow. When the speech clinician works on sounds in words and on words in groups, there is every opportunity to work on phrasing as well. Experiments show that children with articulatory defects often have difficulty with reading. Part of the problem is in the failure to group or phrase words, that is, reading "word by word." Help in phrasing, and practice in grouping words according to thought, can do a great deal to improve the intelligibility of the speaker with articulatory defects.

Intonation or the Melody of Language

Every language has for ordinary, non-emotional communication its own characteristic intonation or melody. This melody plays a strong semantic role in conveying thought. The same words with different intonations change the entire meaning of a sentence.

Stress is one of the modifying factors governing intonation. By changing stress, intonation is always changed, articulation is often changed, and phrasing may be changed. Since one cannot voice anything without intoning the utterance in some way, it is important to teach the intonation that logically belongs to the thought being conveyed.

Intonation depends entirely upon the speaker's thought. It has a pattern, but not a rigid one. A speaker can select his own stresses and intonation, provided they are logical according to his own ideas, and provided the pattern is appropriate to the language being spoken. A speaker who has articulatory defects can do much to improve his fluency by practicing those intonation patterns that give his utterances heightened variety and intelligibility.

ARTICULATORY DISTORTIONS IN THE NORMAL DEVELOPMENT OF SPEECH

There is a normal stage in the early speech development of the child when "baby talk" with its characteristic phonetic distortions is the order of the day. Sometimes, this style of speech is prolonged by over-indulgent parents. Usually, normal maturation or growing older will correct the difficulty.

In a study by Poole (1) involving 140 preschool children, the author states that the fact that sounds are not perfected at the same age by all normal children, is due to multiple variants. These factors are: auditory, kinesthetic or sensory discrimination, motor exercise, and dentition. Poole also found that slightly more than sixty-four per cent of the consonants that appear most often in the words of children, are articulated correctly by them before the age of four and one half years. Further data indicate that thirty-five per cent of the consonants that appear least often in the words of children are not articulated correctly before five and one half years of age.

The following phenomena occur in the speech distortions of normal children: velars and sibilants are distorted most often; omission of single sounds occurs frequently, as in *ittle* for *little;* whole syllables are omitted, as in *ba* for *baby;* substitutions of alveolars for velars occur, as in *dood dirl* for good girl and *tate* for *cake;* assimilation occurs in *gugar* for sugar and *goggie* for doggie; metathesis, the transposing of sounds, occurs in *aks* for *ask* and in *evenlope* for *envelope.*

B. DISORDERS OF ARTICULATION

Definition of Articulatory Disorders

Articulatory disorders may be indicative of various conditions which cause speech difficulties. Defects in articulation are frequently symptomatic of hearing loss, aphasia, cleft palate, cerebral palsy, mental retardation, or foreign accent. In this chapter, however, the authors will limit the term *articulatory defects* to those abnormalities in speech function for which neither medical nor psychological examination has revealed the cause.

Children with articulatory defects usually have comparatively little difficulty in pronouncing vowels. Consonants, on the other hand, present many problems.

Causes of Articulatory Disorders

Parents, physicians, and speech clinicians are anxious to discover some definite organic mouth pathology to explain the child's articulatory problems. Tongue-tie, sluggish velum, abnormally high and arched palate, poorly spaced or missing teeth, are among the possible causes considered. In the majority of cases of articulatory disorders in children, however, no mouth deficiencies are found. Rarely is it necessary to suggest cutting the frenum.

The structural causes for defects in articulation are often overemphasized. Many persons exhibit structural anomalies of the organs of articulation, but have no defects in speech. The chief organ for compensation of deformities of the mouth is the tongue. It is capable of many movements and adjustments which may compensate for many abnormalities. For example, for several of the sounds of speech, one or more alternate mechanical adjustments of articulation may be made. If the speaker cannot use the tip of the tongue to articulate against the alveolar or upper gum ridge, the blade (the part behind the tip) may be used for the alveolar sounds.

Karlin, Youtz, and Kennedy (2) state that the causes of articulatory disorders may be approached from several points of view. First, adequate neurological maturation is necessary for the proper functioning of the articulatory mechanism. Second, pathological conditions such as auditory defects, lack of motor coordination, or the possibility of endocrine disorders must be ruled out. Karlin believes that in some children with defective articulation, the possibility of subclinical endocrine disturbance such as thyroid deficiency or obesity of pituitary origin, may have to be entertained. Third, the authors feel that non-organic environmental factors play a role in molding the child's articulation in speech. Certainly, unfavorable parental attitudes can play a part in preventing proper articulation.

Karlin also found that children with defects in articulation scored low in tests measuring the speed of production of speech, as compared to a control group of children exhibiting normal articulation. Furthermore, children with articulatory disorders showed retardation in their ability to do tasks that required motor speed. It is assumed that neurological maturation, in some areas, may lag behind that of the normal.

In testing hearing in the experimental and control groups, Karlin, Youtz, and Kennedy (2) discovered that the majority of children without articulatory defects demonstrated a superiority of hearing in all frequencies, although both groups possessed adequate auditory acuity. The discrepancy in hearing in the two groups showed itself especially in the high frequencies. It is interesting to note that although the experimental group showed lessened *auditory acuity,* they were superior to the control group in tasks requiring the organization of *visually* attractive materials when the subjects were given unlimited time. In the speech test, children with distorted speech imitated isolated speech sounds surprisingly well, but none of them could combine the sounds into words.

It is possible that disorders of articulation in children are due to retarded growth and development. Although the terms growth and development are often used interchangeably, growth refers to an increase in size, while development means an increase in function or complexity. Usually, these two processes proceed simultaneously, having alternate periods of rapid and slow progress. Sometimes, however, growth may proceed at a normal rate while development may be somewhat retarded. At times, there may be considerable development and little growth. Retardation in either growth or development may be general or it may manifest itself predominantly in some speech organ or system. Distorted speech may be regarded as an index of developmental deficiency or retardation in the speech areas.

It is obvious that the articulation of speech sounds requires both speed and skill in motor ability so far as the speech mechanism is concerned. Many studies of the relationship between motor ability and articulation have been made. Among the more recent ones is that by Jenkins and Lohr (3). Using the *Ozeretsky Tests of Motor Proficiency,* the motor skills of two groups were tested. One group had severe articulatory disorders while the other had no history of speech problems.

The Ozeretsky Tests consisted of batteries which evaluated general static coordination, general dynamic coordination, speed, simultaneous voluntary movement, and *synkinesia* (overflow movement). The experimental group consisted of children whose speech was characterized by poor intelligibility and a number of articulatory errors. They were all first grade children with no physical, mental, or emotional problems. The results indicated that the children with severe articulatory deficiencies had more difficulty in motor proficiency than those without articulatory defects. The implication is that the evaluation of motor ability may be an important factor in diagnosing and planning therapy for children with severe articulatory defects. Jenkins and Lohr (3) concluded by stating that since some children with severe deficits in articulation had high motor proficiency, it is not a contributory factor in every case.

Types of Articulatory Disorders

The most frequent types of articulatory defects are substitutions, distortions, and omissions of sounds. Generally speaking, the most frequently distorted sounds are *s* and *z*. Next in frequency are the consonants θ and ð as in *thin* and *then*, the *l* and *r*, and the *f* and *v* sounds. Substitutions of *t* for *k* and *d* for *g* are also often heard.

Disorders of articulation are classified as follows: *lisping, lalling,* and *other forms of infant perseveration.*

Lisping

The most common type of articulatory defect is the *lisp.* This difficulty is a handicap since the sound *s* occurs more frequently than any other sound in the English language. Any mispronunciation of this sound calls attention to itself frequently and, therefore, interferes with communication.

Pray (4), during her many years as speech clinician, "collected" lisps. She listed sixty-two types of distortion of the sibilant consonant *s*. A lisp in the ordinary sense is limited to distortions of the sound *s*. In a broader sense, however, a lisp may be defined as any mispronunciation of the sibilants *s*, *z*, *ʃ*, *ʒ*, *tʃ*, and *dʒ*. Some speakers distort only one or two of these, the *s* and *z*, while others distort all six sibilant consonants.

The consonant *s* is a high frequency sound which is difficult to record or transmit accurately. There are two methods given for the articulation of the sounds *s* and *z*. These two methods are termed *apical* and *dorsal*.

The apical method is generally preferred. It is shown by Gurren in Figure 31. The point of articulation is the upper gum ridge. The manner of articulation is apical, that is, the tip of the tongue is raised to a position almost touching the upper gum ridge. The sides of the tongue touch the upper side teeth so that no air may escape laterally. The breath passes out through the very narrow passage between the upper gum ridge and the tip of the tongue. The vocal cords do not vibrate. The result is a voiceless, hissing, fricative consonant.

In the dorsal method of articulating the sound *s*, the point of articulation is the same as in the first description, the upper gum ridge. The manner of articulation is, however, very different from the first. In dorsal articulation, the tip of the tongue is down behind the lower teeth, and the front of the tongue, the part behind the tip, articulates close to the gum ridge. The resulting sound is a fricative, voiceless, hissing consonant somewhat less clear than the one produced by the apical method. There is some danger in using the dorsal position of the tongue for the sound *s* since it often results in a muffled, indistinct sibilant. On the other hand, if the speaker has marked dental malocclusions or abnormal jaw structure, it may be necessary to teach the dorsal articulation of the sound *s*.

The sound *z* is produced in the same way as the sound *s*, except that the vocal cords vibrate to produce the sound *z*. The sounds *ʃ* and *ʒ* are produced by placing the tip of the tongue almost touching the upper gum ridge in a place a little farther back than the point of articulation for the sound *s*. The manner of articulation is similar to that for *s* and *z*. The sound *ʃ* is voice-

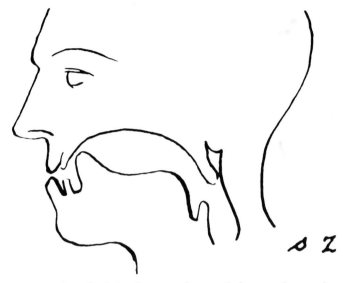

Figure 31. Apical method for the articulation of the sounds *s* and *z*. From Louise Gurren's *A Comparison on a Phonetic Basis of the Two Chief Languages of the Americas, English and Spanish*. Ph.D. Thesis, New York University, 1955. (Illustration by F. Manopoli.)

less, and the sound ʒ is voiced. The consonants *t*ʃ and *d*ʒ are made up of two sounds, *t* + ʃ and *d* + ʒ respectively as is indicated in Table IV, page 59. The tongue touches the upper gum ridge for *t*, is quickly lowered slightly and raised to a position a little further back than it is for *s* to articulate the sound ʃ. The sound *t*ʃ is voiceless while the sound *d*ʒ, produced in the same way, is voiced.

Types of Lisp

One of the common types of lisp is the *lingual protrusion lisp*. As was previously explained, the clear *s* is produced by placing the tongue almost touching the upper gum ridge. The child who has a lingual protrusion lisp places the tongue between the teeth to say the sound *s*. The resulting sound is close to the θ in *thin*. Thus, the child says *thikth* for *six*. This type of lisp is often caused by infant perseveration or "baby talk." This lisp may also be caused by malocclusions of the teeth and by missing upper front teeth.

Another common type of lisp is the *lateral emission lisp*. The resulting sound produced is a whispered *l* since in this type of lisp the speaker, instead of having the sides of the tongue raised to touch the upper side teeth, lowers the tongue on either or both sides so that the air escapes laterally instead of from the center of the mouth. The result is a very indistinct sound which detracts from the effectiveness of communication.

Another type of lisp is the *dental* form. In this case, the tip of the tongue is placed near the upper teeth instead of close to the upper gum ridge. The resulting sound is not so indistinct as the lateral emission lisp, but it is noticeably different from the alveolar *s*.

Less frequently encountered are the *inverted s* and the *nasal emission lisps*. In the former, the speaker curls back the tip of the tongue almost in the position for the sound *r*. The breath passes over the space between the rolled tip of the tongue and the front of the hard palate. The resulting sound is a very indistinct voiceless consonant, similar to a whispered *r*. The nasal emission type of lisp is most frequently heard from the child with a cleft palate or with an unusually high, pointed arch in the roof of the mouth. It may also be found in children with faulty control of the uvula. This sound is formed by placing the tip of the tongue on the alveolar ridge, thus preventing the air from passing out through the mouth. The sound thus produced is similar to a whispered *n*. This type of lisp causes low intelligibility in communication.

Another type of distortion is the substitution of the sound ʃ for *s*. In this type of articulation, the tongue is placed in a position farther back toward the hard palate than it is for the sound *s*.

Less frequent, but causing very low intelligibility in communication, is the omission of the sound *s* in all positions. Children with hearing loss in the high frequency range will omit the *s* in their speech.

Lalling

Another type of articulatory distortion is *lalling*. This is usually described as the substitution of the sound *w* for the consonants *l* and *r*. Thus, *little* becomes *wittiw*, and red rose becomes *wed wose*. A less frequent substitution for *l* is the sound *j*. Children who have this type of baby talk say *yike* for *like* and *pyay* for *play*.

Other Forms of Infant Perseveration

In general, many of the articulatory difficulties referred to previously are due to lack of maturation. A child of five or six years of age should be able to distinguish between the velar and alveolar consonants, that is between the *g* and the *d*, and the *k* and the *t* sounds. Children who do not distinguish between these sounds in their speech, say *dive* for *give* and *tan* for *can*.

Another form of distortion is the substitution of the labio-dentals *f* and *v* for the dental sounds θ as in *thin* and ᵟ as in *then*. This type of distortion results in the substitution of *fin* for *thin* and *vis* for *this*.

It is possible that immature eight-year-olds may lisp and have all the other sound substitutions of infant speech. Some of the sound substitutions last into adult life if they are not corrected in early school years. Infant perseveration in speech is a distinct disadvantage socially and vocationally, since it gives the impression of immaturity, even if the speaker is emotionally and professionally mature.

DIAGNOSIS OF ARTICULATORY DISORDERS

Before treating the child, it is important to diagnose the nature, degree, and possible cause of the defect. As defined in this text, these difficulties are not due to organic causes, such as: hearing loss, mental retardation, or other physical or intellectual handicaps. One must consider the factor of environmental influences as a vital part of the child's speech development. Over-protective parents may cause slow emotional maturation in the child, a definite factor in articulatory defects.

It is essential to become acquainted with the child and the parents before administering any formal kind of articulation test. This may be done by first interviewing the parents and child together. Later, the speech clinician can talk to them separately, unless it is difficult to see the child alone. During the initial interview, the speech consultant can accumulate pertinent facts as to the family background of the child. Questions regarding brothers and sisters, schooling, recreational preferences, and playmates may be asked. If the child is incapable of answering, the mother may supply the details. Answers to these questions provide the necessary background that helps the speech clinician to become acquainted with the child. Health and school records are also essential for an adequate diagnosis.

Two methods should be employed by the speech clinician to evaluate the articulatory disorders of the child. The *picture method* coupled with *listening to connected speech* provide an insight into the child's problems.

The picture method is useful to evaluate the articulation of the sounds of English. This is of importance regardless of whether the child knows how to read. One must take an inventory of the sounds of the language spoken by the youngster. The picture method forms the first procedure to use in uncovering articulatory defects. Used alone, however, it is inadequate for a complete evaluation of the child's speech problems. Sounds may be reasonably clear in isolation and in single words, but they may be indistinct to the point of unintelligibility in connected speech. The second method of listening to connected speech is, therefore, essential.

In order to elicit more than single words, it is necessary to use questions that relate to the child's interests and background. If, for example, he mentions watching television as one of his favorite pastimes, he may be asked to describe his favorite program. Questions must be concrete. If the child is hesitant, the speech clinician must be a patient listener. If a child seems unable to answer one question in connected speech, after waiting a suitable time, the clinician should ask another, based on a different topic. For example, most young children know the stories, *The Three Bears* and *Red Riding Hood*. They may be asked to tell the story. Gurren finds this kind of stimulus quite effective for young children.

While the child is talking, it is advisable to record mental notes, rather than to write too much. The use of the International

Phonetic Alphabet is an excellent way to take down observations regarding the articulation of children.

It is important to record both correct as well as incorrect articulation in both single words and in connected speech. Some children are disconcerted by having the listener take copious notes while they are speaking. After the child has left, the clinician can fill in and complete the records.

The speech clinician should provide a variety of diagnostic material. This should include books that contain pictures of objects that represent all the sounds of English. Consonants should be tested in various positions in the word or sentence. Sommers (5) describes an articulation test that was used for his study. This test, developed by E. T. McDonald, classifies the consonants according to *arrestors* and *releasors* of syllables. This approach is a departure from the *initial, medial,* and *final* classifications of consonants according to the position of the sound in the word. The releasors and arrestors are those consonants that initiate or end a syllable. Since a syllable is a group of sounds that are voiced in one impulse, such sound groupings are important for testing articulation. It has been noted that children with disorders of articulation often say sounds in isolation accurately, but have difficulty in saying the same sounds in combination.

The purpose of an articulatory test is threefold. First, it should provide a means of identification and localization of the sound or sounds that are defective. Second, it should be able to give an analysis of the deviations in articulation that cause the distortion. Third, it should provide an estimate of the degree of the deviation. In general, it may be said that disorders of articulation are the result of inaccurate functioning of the articulators.

The child's behavior and reactions should be noted during the interview with the speech clinician. In addition to pictures and books, the subject should be provided with three dimensional materials in the form of toys. The speech clinician can also make use of objects in the office such as, the telephone, the pencils, and the desk blotter. In this case, the child is asked to name and tell the use of the object. Gurren has seen children who were at first reluctant to talk, speak quite willingly into a telephone.

Many of them enjoy handling three dimensional objects and, consequently, are more willing to communicate orally when they are examining toys or other objects in the office. It cannot be overemphasized that diagnosis is a continuing process and that one or two interviews cannot suffice for an accurate and complete speech evaluation. In fact, more complete diagnosis takes place during treatment.

During the diagnostic interviews, the parents will be most anxious to know the clinician's opinion of the prognosis. Most articulatory defects are remediable, given a child with normal intelligence, reasonable emotional stability, and no marked organic handicap. The tongue is a remarkable adjuster. It can often modify and improve articulation, given training and practice. While it is often unwise to predict complete correction, the parents can be encouraged to believe that, with time, and with their help at home, the child's articulation should be very much improved.

TREATMENT OF ARTICULATORY DISORDERS

It is important to state and to re-state the fact that while a sound unit may be examined separately, one must always bear in mind that it has to be built back into the rapid and continuous synergy of muscle movement necessary for connected speech.

The statement has been made by Van Riper (6) that more than seventy per cent of all speech defects are articulatory and that they are usually treated haphazardly. The treatment of speech disorders is both a science and an art. The speech clinician, therefore, has to acquire the exact facts about the scientific aspect of his profession. After years of practice, he may learn to modify and apply these facts intelligently.

One of the most important aspects in the treatment of disorders of articulation is parent counseling. Individual interviews combined with group meetings are exceedingly important. The speech consultant should acquaint parents with the normal speech development of the child and should point out to them definite, practical ways of helping the child improve his articulation. It is essential to mention that too much stress and constant correction are to be avoided. The speech clinician should ask the parents to supplement his work by using speech games and jingles that will be helpful and enjoyable for home use.

Methods and Materials in the
Treatment of Articulatory Disorders

The speech consultant, in a series of planned meetings with the child, should provide sequential, developmental lessons in articulation. All materials should be based on the age and background of the child, and should be varied to keep interest alive. The motto, "little and often," is useful in many cases. Therefore, speech lessons should be as frequent as possible, but not of too long duration. At the beginning, for some children, fifteen minutes should suffice. As the child progresses, and feels the need for further improvement, the lessons may be increased to twenty or even thirty minutes for group work.

The speech clinician should have a thorough knowledge of the sounds of English, and of how the sounds are formed. He should also be familiar with the phonetic structure of language and with the role of each aspect of the structure in improving intelligibility in speech. Every meeting with the child or group of children should provide for sound analysis, and application of sounds in words, in phrases, and in connected speech. Assignments should be given to the child to practice at home with the parents.

It is essential to remember that children vary greatly in improvement of articulation. Intelligence, physical structure and performance of the speech organs, aptitude, and emotional attitude toward speech are important factors for accelerating or decreasing the speed of improvement. In any case, no lasting correction takes place quickly. Clear articulation in connected speech must become automatic before the speech consultant can feel that the child's difficulties have been overcome.

Summary of Techniques in Treatment

The first step in the improvement of articulation is *ear training,* so that the child may be able to differentiate or discriminate between the incorrect sound that he makes and the proper one that should be used in its place. The second step after auditory stimulation has been enhanced is the *phonetic placement method,* or the description of how the sound is formed. The third step is to provide *strengthening of the sound* in isolation through practice material. Lastly, the speech clinician should provide for the *transition from the isolated sound to the use of the sound in words and in connected speech.*

The child must be made to recognize that there is a goal for him to reach through motivation on the part of the speech clinician. The greater the number of stimuli used to learn the new pattern, the better will be the results. Combined auditory, visual, motor, and kinesthetic stimuli will do much more to set a new pattern than will a single stimulus. While it is important to hold the attention of the child by judicious variety of material, it is equally important to avoid presenting a hodge-podge of stimuli. The importance of careful planning of each meeting cannot be overemphasized. In planning lessons and preparing materials, it is usually helpful to work with the sound in the initial position first, then in the final position, and last in the medial position. Blends of consonants may then be practiced.

Although it is essential to make the child aware of his disorder, it is important to avoid embarrassing him. The child must not feel resentment toward speech training. In general, the speech reminders and corrections should take place at definite and appropriate times, both at meetings with the speech clinician and in the home. When the child is at play, or when the family is gathered for a social evening at home, constant nagging about speech becomes inappropriate. Since speech is a form of behavior, a total reaction pattern including methods of working with the child's speech must be carefully considered and planned. Only in this way can the child achieve the long-range goal of heightened intelligibility in communication through improvement in articulation of speech.

REFERENCES

(1) Poole, I.: A Study of the Development of Consonant Sounds in Young Children's Speech. Unpublished Doctoral Thesis. Ann Arbor, University of Michigan, 1934.

(2) Karlin, I. W., Youtz, A. C., and Kennedy, L: Distorted Speech in Young Children. *Am. J. Dis. Child.*, 59:1203, June, 1940.

(3) Jenkins, E., and Lohr, F. E.: Panel Discussion. New York, American Speech and Hearing Association Convention, November, 1962.

(4) Pray, S.: *Directions for the Production of English Consonants.* New York, Author's publication, 1929.

(5) Sommers, R. K.: Factors in the Effectiveness of Mothers Trained to Aid in Speech Correction. *J. Speech Hearing Disorders,* 27:178, May, 1962.

(6) Van Riper, C.: *Speech Correction; Principles and Methods.* New York, Prentice-Hall, 1963.

Chapter 9

APHASIAS IN CHILDREN

HISTORY

Gall, about 1800, was the first to suggest that the brain was composed of "organs" which control the "vital and moral faculties of man." Although Gall was a phrenologist, he was not a charlatan. He believed that speech and memory of words were situated in the frontal lobes. He was one of the first to believe in cortical localization of function.

Broca, in 1861, concluded from a study of pathological specimens, that the inferior frontal gyrus (convolution) in the brain was the seat of articulate speech. He described *aphemia,* or motor aphasia, as the language disturbance resulting from a lesion in the inferior frontal gyrus of the left cerebral hemisphere. Broca's work centered largely on the expressive or motor language problems and this language defect became known as *Broca's aphasia* (see Figure 17, page 69).

Wernicke, in 1873, described an auditory center in the superior temporal gyrus. In his now famous treatise, *The Aphasic Symptom Complex,* he introduced the concept of sensory centers in this gyrus and demonstrated that the superior temporal convolution was the site for the reception of auditory impulses at the level of comprehension. Wernicke's work was so widely accepted that the superior temporal gyrus became known as Wernicke's area. Thus, plentiful free speech characterized by errors due to loss of normal auditory control, associated with a lack of understanding of spoken words, became known as sensory or *Wernicke's aphasia.*

Wernicke also described an aphasia caused by a defect in the conducting mechanism between temporal centers and other cortical areas. He also described total aphasia in which both the auditory receptor center together with the motor centers are involved.

Hughlings Jackson (1), in 1879, was the first to emphasize that the problems in the understanding of aphasia had important psychological aspects. He believed in the dynamic behavior of the individual and formulated the term "propositional" speech. He defined this term as being a relationship among words that brings a new meaning, not by the addition of separate meanings of each word used, but rather, by their modifications, one upon the other. "Single words are meaningless and so is any unrelated succession of words. The unit of speech is not the word, but the proposition formed by the interaction of all the words used." The formulation of a proposition is a psychological function as is the understanding of speech. The aphasic individual lacks this ability to propositionalize." Jackson felt that emotional and automatic speech are not propositional speech, for he observed that although many of his patients could use automatic speech, they were unable to express a proposition. Furthermore, Jackson demonstrated that differently situated cortical lesions affect different elements of speech.

Jackson was the great "nonlocalizationist." He argued against the localization of speech areas, such as that of Broca's area. He felt that there were no narrowly defined areas in the cortex as centers for language development. Rather, he introduced a psychological approach stressing the dissolution of language behavior in individuals with aphasia. He formulated concepts of higher and lower levels of behavior, wherein the loss of voluntary language frees the involuntary acts. Jackson gave one an appreciation of the close relationship between thought and language and the observation that they were not one and the same. He also felt that *paraphasia* may be a purely functional symptom of reduced efficiency of the apparatus of speech.

Charcot, in 1883, introduced the concept of a writing center and an ideation center. The ideation center was believed to be an integrating force for all other centers of cortical activity. Charcot was the first to observe differences in behavior existing between individuals suffering from the same or similar neurological disturbances. Thus, he postulated the existence of different kinds of individuals. Some he felt were visual-minded, while others were auditory-minded. Therefore, a defect in the visual center of a visual-minded person caused greater disability than a similar defect in the visual center of an auditory-minded person.

Freud, in 1891, insisted on the compatibility of the localization approach with the functional approach in the problem of aphasia. He considered all aphasias to originate from interruptions of conducting mechanisms or associations. According to Freud, aphasia is due to a lesion of those association fibers that meet in a nodal point called a center. An organic genesis of the symptom does not negate the possibility that the same symptom remains subject to physiological and psychological laws.

In 1906, Marie, one of Broca's students, stated that speech is an intellectual function and that aphasia is associated with general intellectual deficiency and a special language deficit. Marie felt that there was only one kind of aphasia, namely, Wernicke's aphasia. He claimed that Broca's aphasia is Wernicke's aphasia plus *anarthria*. Marie localized all lesions in a quadrilateral space consisting of the basal ganglia, internal capsule, external capsule, and the insula.

Head, in 1910, described aphasia as a disorder of symbolic thinking and expression. He believed in four types of aphasias:

1. Verbal aphasia—exemplified by defective word formation.
2. Syntactical aphasia—a lack of coherence and a tendency to talk jargon.
3. Nominal aphasia—defective use of nouns, both spoken and written.
4. Semantic aphasia—deficient comprehension of the full significance of words and phrases.

During the early twentieth century, Goldstein (2) formulated the concept that the aphasic has lost the capacity to demonstrate abstract behavior. The aphasic is able to comprehend and express only the concrete and more realistic attitudes.

INTRODUCTION

The term "phasia" is a combining form used to denote speech. The word "aphasia" literally means "without speech." A good definition of *aphasia* is given by Fulton (3) in Howell's *Textbook of Physiology.* "The term aphasia means literally the loss of the power of speech, but the term is now used to include any marked interference with the ability either to use or to comprehend symbolic expression of ideas by spoken or written words or by gestures." Aphasia is not an absence of speech, but rather a lack of language communication mediated through speech. Head (4) refers to speech as symbolic behavior and describes aphasia as a disorder of symbolic formulation and expression.

Aphasia is a language disorder associated with brain damage. It is characterized by loss or impairment in the use of spoken or written symbols for the formulation, reception, or transmission of ideas. *Dysphasia* is a term used to designated a milder degree of such a disturbance.

There are three chief classifications in which the function of speech is disturbed or non-existent. First, there are patients in whom there is an abnormality of the higher intellectual functions. The condition may be congential as in the case of idiots; inflammatory as in acquired dementia; or psychiatric as in the case of hysteria. Such patients are speechless but they are not aphasic.

Second, there are cases in which the higher intellectual functions are intact, but in which there is paralysis or incoordination of certain groups of muscles required for articulation. Such cases of speech impairment are found in paralysis of the palate or tongue, bulbar paralysis or disease of the cerebellum. These patients have dysarthria but are not aphasic.

Third, there are cases in which there are no paralyses of the peripheral organs of speech. Rather, the patient exhibits a language disorder in the areas of symbolization, in comprehension, and in reproduction of concepts whenever attempting to use conventional spoken or written symbols. It is this disability that is termed aphasia.

To be exact, one should differentiate between *speech* and *language.* Language is a psychic process centered in the cortex, which expresses thoughts and ideas. Military communication through semaphore and the manual alphabet of deaf mutes is language just as much as verbal communication. Speech is the expression of feelings and ideas through sounds and spoken words. It is the verbal means of communication and may be regarded as both a tool and a manifestation of language. In general usage, the terms speech and language are interchangeable, and in this chapter these terms will be so used.

The time-honored division of aphasia into motor and sensory types is a pathological classification. It is legitimate pathologically to distinguish efferent from afferent impairment of function. As far as speech is concerned, it is doubtful whether a pure case of either motor or sensory aphasia ever exists. It can be stated, however, that lesions toward the anterior part of the speech region are predominantly motor or expressive, while lesions in the posterior portion of the speech area are predominantly sensory or receptive.

ANATOMICAL CONSIDERATIONS

Differences of opinion still exist as to the specificity of functions of certain areas of the brain. If placed on a continuum, one end of the scale would represent an attitude of pinpoint specificity of function, localized in circumscribed areas called cortical centers. The opposite extremity would represent an attitude of almost complete equality of function in all parts of the cortex, the nonlocalization viewpoint. The consensus today is that there is specialization of function of certain areas of the cortex, but at the same time there must be an over-all integration.

Before discussing the problem of aphasia in children, one must familiarize himself with the regional anatomy of the brain related to speech as well as with the levels of cortical functions and their abnormalities.

The normal activity of the central nervous system depends upon the interaction of two systems, the sensory and the motor. The sensory, or receptive, component of speech consists of comprehending spoken or written language, i.e., spoken words or written symbols. The motor, or expressive, component of speech consists in the ability to express words or written symbols. In the development of speech, associations are formed between verbal sounds or words, and meaning. Thus, associations are established in specialized areas of the cerebral cortex. These areas are depicted in Brodman's cytoarchitectonic fields of the human cerebral cortex. In 1909, Brodman separated forty-seven areas of

the cortex said to be histologically distinct. Only those related
to speech will be enumerated here.

The sensory or receptive speech areas, like all sensory cerebral
representation, is located posterior to the Rolandic and Sylvian
fissures. Wernicke's auditory area in the superior temporal gyrus
is area 41 (see Figure 32). It also occupies the floor of the
Sylvian fissure and is surrounded by the psychoauditory zone,
area 42. Area 37, immediately anterior to the occipital lobe, is
the language formulation area, where the child lays down engrams for the proper arrangement of words into sentences. The
visual cortex surrounding the calcarine fissure is area 17. The
visual word area is in the angular gyrus, area 39.

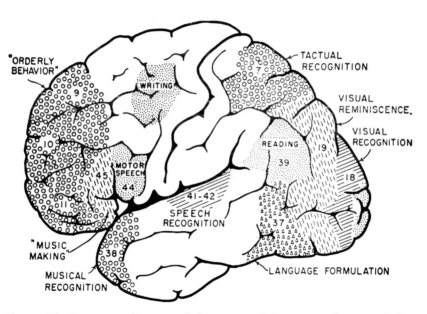

Figure 32. Composite diagram of the supposed "association" areas of the
human cerebral cortex. From C. T. Morgan and E. Stellar's *Physiological
Psychology*, 2nd Ed., copyright 1950. Courtesy of the McGraw-Hill Book
Company, Inc., New York, New York. Used by permission.

The motor or expressive area is located at the posterior end
of the inferior frontal convolution. It is area 44 and is known
as Broca's convolution. Broca's area is not the direct cortical

representation of the muscles of speech, but it lies just anterior to it. The writing area is part of the cheirokinesthetic area and is situated above Broca's area.

It is evident from these observations that the receptive areas for speech are situated in the posterior part of the cortex, while the motor areas are primarily associated with the anterior part. It is also evident that the area of the cortex devoted to the reception of speech is much larger than that occupied with its expression. The apparatus for speech presents itself as a continuous cortical area in the left cerebral hemisphere. It extends between the termination of the acoustic and optic nerves and the origin of the motor tracts for the muscles serving articulation.

FORMS OF APHASIA

The speech defects most commonly observed in aphasia are either predominantly motor or predominantly sensory. In the predominantly motor form, the greatest disturbance is in the ability to express ideas in speech and/or in writing. Lesions centered in the inferior frontal convolution of the left cerebral hemisphere cause loss of speech. This area, Broca's gyrus, is, therefore, the cortical center in which are laid down engrams representing the memory of how to make movements of the vocal organs for the purpose of speaking. Broca's aphasia is thus a form of *apraxia.* The individual has forgotten how to make the movements necessary for speech.

Lesions centered in the superior temporal convolution produce predominantly sensory disturbances. This is Wernicke's aphasia, or *word deafness,* in which the individual cannot comprehend spoken symbols. With lesions in the angular gyrus, the speech disturbance involves chiefly the visual elements. The individual cannot read or recognize pictures. This disability is called *alexia* or *word blindness.* Writing may be involved although articulation is intact. Lesions in the posterior part of the second frontal convolution just anterior to the motor area of the arm produce *agraphia* or inability to write. In localized temporal lobe lesions such as abscess formation, *anomia* or *optic aphasia* may be present. In more extensive temporal lobe lesions, the person may exhibit *paraphasia* or *jargon aphasia* in which the individual is voluble, but employs words unsuitable to express his meaning.

Less commonly observed are the *amnesic* and *semantic* aphasias. In amnesic aphasia, there is difficulty in the evocation or recall of well-known objects. In semantic aphasia, the individual has little difficulty in speaking or understanding words, but the general meaning of what is heard or read escapes him. In some cases, all language processes, both motor and sensory, are severely disturbed. This is commonly referred to as *global* aphasia and is due to a lesion in the left supramarginal gyrus.

LEVELS OF CORTICAL FUNCTION

Teitelbaum (5) and Nielsen (6) have shown that certain cortical functions often referred to as higher, or as occurring at a higher cortical level, are dependent upon a more complex integrative activity than those cortical functions which are referred to as lower, or as occurring at a lower cortical level. The development of language function also follows an order of increasing cortical complexity.

Figure 33 traces the increased complexity of language in the

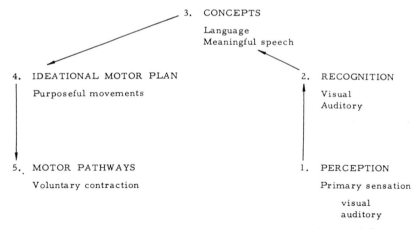

Figure 33. Diagram showing the developmental levels of cortical function. From Isaac W. Karlin's Aphasias in Children, *American Journal of Diseases of Children*, 87:752, 1954. Courtesy of American Medical Association, Chicago, Illinois.

growing child. The infant at first receives sensory impulses such as sound and visual stimulation. He then develops a perception or an awareness of these sensory stimuli. These impulses end in the cortex at the first level, called by Orton (7) the "arrival platform."

The child next develops recognition, which is a cortical function on the next higher level above that of perception. At this second level, the child acquires the ability to recognize various objects and symbols. Memory constellations are formed which are capable of recall.

As the child becomes older, some of these functions are further refined at yet a higher level and one enters the realm of concept formulation or symbolization. Thus, language is elaborated. All the above mentioned levels are sensory.

In the motor sphere, there is a similar arrangement in order of increasing integrative complexity. At the lowest level, motor pathways are developed through the ability to contract striated muscle voluntarily. At the second level, there is the ability to perform planned, purposeful movements of varying degrees of complexity. Finally, at the highest level, there is the ability to express meaningful speech and language.

When there is a disturbance at any of these sensory or motor levels, disorders result as shown in Figure 34. The right side of the figure indicates the sensory involvement, while the left side depicts the motor pathology.

Loss of primary perception, cortical blindness or deafness, results from a lesion at the first level, on the sensory side. At the second sensory level, visual or auditory agnosia takes place. Receptive aphasia, or loss of concept formation, develops at the third level.

Lesions at the first level on the motor side result in anarthria. Apraxia develops at the second level of motor involvement. Finally, at the third level, motor aphasia is in evidence.

CLASSIFICATION

Aphasia is a defect in symbolic language due to cerebral pathology. In the adult, aphasia signifies an acquired loss of a previously existing function. In the child, aphasia denotes a

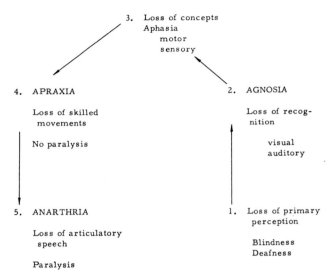

3. Loss of concepts
Aphasia
   motor
   sensory

4. APRAXIA

   Loss of skilled
   movements

   No paralysis

5. ANARTHRIA

   Loss of articulatory
   speech

   Paralysis

2. AGNOSIA

   Loss of recog-
   nition

      visual
      auditory

1. Loss of primary
   perception

   Blindness
   Deafness

Figure 34. Diagram showing the disturbances produced at various levels of cortical function. From Isaac W. Karlin's Aphasias in Children, *American Journal of Diseases of Children*, 87:752, 1954. Courtesy of the American Medical Association, Chicago, Illinois.

cerebral form of language dysfunction which may be either acquired or congenital.

Congenital aphasia means that the brain damage is present at birth. It may be due to an aplasia, a defect in development, or a delay in maturation of certain cortical areas in the prenatal period. It may also be due to some noxious factors that damaged these areas either prenatally or at birth.

Conrad, working chiefly in the field of configurational psychology, believes that in aphasia, verbal expression is inhibited or precluded by blocking mechanisms which occur during the *vorgestalt,* or those mental processes which take place immediately prior to the exteriorization of words in speech and writing. A similar view is expressed by Critchley (8). He speaks of *preverbitum* which may be defined as the mental activity which immediately precedes speech. The clinical character of the aphasia depends upon the depth at which the preverbital blockage occurs.

Aphasia in children is a controversial subject. Some investigators deny the existence of congenital aphasia unless there is severe bilateral brain damage. Some object to the use of the term aphasia for children who never had speech, since aphasia implies the loss of a previously existing function. Others feel that aphasia in children implies an unusual language disorder.

While theoretically one may postulate that congenital aphasia does not exist as an entity, clinically there is no doubt that there are children with severe language disabilities who are misdiagnosed as cases of deafness, emotional disorder, or mental retardation. Although there are differences between aphasia in the adult and aphasia in the child, aphasia is still a good generic term since it denotes a cerebral form of language dysfunction. Karlin (9) has proposed the following classification:

Aphasias in Children

A. *Acquired*
1. Acute—due to infections, convulsions, migraine
2. Subacute — due to abscess, tumor
3. Chronic—due to trauma, hemorrhage

B. *Congenital*
1. Speech Aphasias
   *a. Verbal-Auditory Agnosia (word deafness)
   **b. Motor Aphasia (dysphasia)
2. Visual Aphasias
   *a. Alexia (word blindness)
   **b. Agraphia

*Sensory
**Motor

One must be aware of the fact that it is the site of the brain involvement rather than the pathological nature of the lesion that determines the symptom complex of aphasia.

The acquired aphasias are comparatively rare. They all have two points in common that differentiate them from the congenital aphasias. First, they are secondary to brain pathology. They are the result of infection, tumor, or cerebral vascular accident. Second, all acquired aphasias present neurological signs or have laboratory evidence of brain pathology.

In the acute acquired type, a marked transient aphasia may follow convulsions. The aphasia may last for a few days or disappear in a few hours. Temporary aphasia may also follow an attack of migraine.

The subacute types of aphasia are the language disturbances that the child may develop as a result of brain tumor or brain abscess. The speech and language disturbances are not as dramatic as in the acute type and are frequently overlooked. Here, one is dealing with a sick, apathetic, and morose child. Not much attention is paid to the speech and language disturbance. A child six to seven years of age may show complete mutism. An older child of ten to twelve years of age, may show hesitancy in speech, distorted speech, a "telegram" style of speech, or the speech picture seen in adult aphasics. Once the underlying pathology is removed, recovery from aphasia is good. Most patients recover in about four weeks.

In the chronic type, the symptomatology resembles that of the aphasias seen in the adult. Here, the aphasia is usually the result of some cerebral vascular accident. Children with cerebral palsy must be differentiated from this group, since they present their own characteristic speech problems.

THE CONGENITAL APHASIAS

Congenital aphasia, or primary aphasia, presents a much more difficult problem than the acquired types. In congenital aphasia, one is discussing a child who presents failure in the development of language function without history or neurological signs of brain disease or brain injury. Failure to develop language may be due to mental deficiency, deafness, or severe emotional disturbances (psychoses), but these children present special problems of their own and should not be considered aphasic.

Congenital Verbal-Auditory Agnosia
(Word Deafness)

The onset of speech in children usually occurs at about eighteen months of age and is earlier in girls than in boys. The absence of speech in a child two or two and one-half years of age should be considered abnormal. Mental retardation, hearing disabilities, and audimutitas should be considered as possible causes for the delay in the development of speech.

There are cases of delayed speech, however, which cannot be explained on the basis of the three above mentioned causes. Congenital verbal-auditory agnosia (congenital word deafness) has to be considered in such cases. Karlin (10) has outlined the clinical features of congenital verbal-auditory agnosia as follows:

1. The child does not talk or has only limited speech. This is always the initial and outstanding sign. It is the child's speech that the parents are primarily concerned about when they take him to the physician. The child of three or four years of age may have no speech at all, or an older one of six years of age may have limited or distorted speech. His speech may also lack stress and intonation.
2. The child appears to be mentally normal.
3. Physical, including neurological, examination is normal.
4. There is a negative history of injury and illness.
5. The child's hearing is the crux of the problem. Classically, the child has normal or adequate hearing when tested with the audiometer, but is unable to comprehend words by the auditory route. In some cases, psychogalvanic skin-resistance audiometry may have to be used to substantiate the diagnosis.

At first, the parents are certain that the child is able to hear. At the child grows older, it becomes evident that he is deaf to speech, and yet is able to hear sounds. It soon appears that the limited speech which the child does acquire is through lip reading. A better understanding of this problem can be had if we realize that in the development of speech, granted a normal intellectual endowment, hearing and speech form a closely interrelated function.

The normal anatomy and physiology of the auditory pathway so essential for speech development is grossly shown in Figure 35. The cochlear division of the auditory nerve arises from the cells of the ganglion of the cochlea of the inner ear and passes into the medulla. Reaching the lower portion of the pons, the fibers divide, one portion going to the dorsal, the other to the ventral, cochlear nuclei. The fibers issuing from these nuclei later unite and ascend as the lateral lemniscus to terminate in the medial geniculate body. Fibers arising from the medial geniculate body form the auditory radiation and ascend in the posterior limb of the internal capsule to terminate in the temporal lobe of the cortex. The primary center where the auditory im-

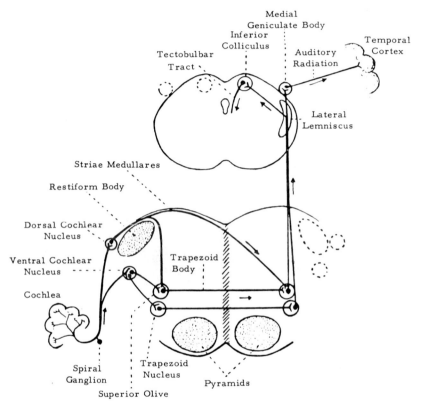

Figure 35. Diagram of the auditory pathway. From Charles Best and Norman Taylor's *The Physiological Basis of Medical Practice* (in part after Gray). From Isaac W. Karlin's Aphasias in Children, *American Journal of Diseases of Children*, 87:752, 1954. Courtesy of the American Medical Association, Chicago, Illinois.

pulse arrives is in the transverse temporal gyrus of Heschl, lying in the floor of the Sylvian fissure. This is the audito-sensory area, or the site of primary perception. Here the fundamental auditory sensations of intensity, quality, and pitch are appreciated. The impulse then travels to the adjacent superior temporal convolution or Wernicke's area. This is the audito-psychic area where there occur the analysis and the interpretation of auditory sensations and their integration into more complex perception. Here occurs the recognition of sounds in general and of language in particular.

Goldstein (2) states that the integrity of Heschl's region guarantees the simple acoustic perceptions, while the integrity of the wider field of Wernicke's area is necessary for perception of the more complex acoustic phenomena of perception of language. Nielsen (11) states that impulses received by the first transverse gyrus of Heschl do not enter consciousness, while those received by Wernicke's area result in recognition of language at a conscious level. Thus, Nielsen calls Heschl's area the site of primary perception and Wernicke's area the site of primary identification.

In the adult, a loss or disturbance in the comprehension of language is known as aphasia. In the child, however, many terms have been used to designate word deafness. Ewing (12) uses the term aphasia although some of his children had high frequency deafness. This might explain the language difficulties that they presented. Others use the term congenital or infantile aphasia. Yet, many investigators object to the use of the term congenital aphasia since in the child, one is not dealing with the loss of a previously existing function but with a failure in the development of a function. To meet this objection, Nance (13) suggests the use of the term ideopathic language retardation. Another term which has been used to describe these cases is psychic deafness in children. Froeschels (14) points out that the term psychic deafness in children is misleading since it may be confused with hysterical deafness or with deafness due to other emotional or psychological factors. Inasmuch as congenital word deafness is not a psychogenic disturbance, Froeschels proposes the term central deafness. Nielsen (6), from his studies of pathological specimens in adults, regards word deafness as being on a lower level than aphasia and groups it under agnosia. Agnosia is a disturbance of recognition or identification, while aphasia is the loss of the recognition of the significance of the word. For children with word deafness, Nielsen uses the term congenital verbal imperception.

While the language or verbal defect is the initial and outstanding external disorder, it is the internal, cortical auditory defect for language that is the actual disorder. Taking Nielsen's view into consideration, Karlin (10) believes a good term for word deafness in the child is congenital verbal-auditory agnosia. This term localizes the defect to the cortical hearing and speech areas.

Concerning the pathogenesis of word deafness, one can only speculate upon the underlying pathology. Worster-Drought and Allen (15) believe that the probable cause is an aplasia of the post-temporal cerebral cortex. They state that since each auditory nerve is connected with both temporal lobes, the defect has to be bilateral. Nielsen (11), from his studies with adults, states that many cases are on record showing that patients with word deafness have a lesion in the middle third of the first temporal convolution on the major side. Best and Taylor (16) state that the audito-psychic area is mainly unilateral, situated on the left side in right-handed individuals. Orton (7) states that neurologists are agreed that a lesion in one brain hemisphere, provided it be the dominant one, is sufficient to cause disorders of spoken and written language. Karlin's (17) theory that stuttering may be due to a delay in, or a lack of, myelinization of cortical speech areas may also be applicable to congenital word deafness.

Congenital Motor Aphasia (Expressive Aphasia)

Congenital motor aphasia is a more infrequent disorder than congenital word deafness. These children do not speak at all or make primitive sounds. They demonstrate some understanding of speech and do not exhibit the auditory inattention characteristic of children with sensory aphasia.

Alexia (Congenital Word Blindness)

The general term reading disability includes a wide variety of clinical entities of apparently different etiologies. A great deal has been said about psychological or emotional factors responsible for reading disabilities. Beginning with Hippocrates or shortly before, all diseases of unknown etiology had been ascribed to emotions. The role of emotions is especially difficult to evaluate. Many individuals are in the midst of an emotional upset, just getting over one, or about to have one. There can be little doubt, however, that the course, or at least the degree, of reading disability is in large measure influenced by the patient's emotional reactions.

Congenital word blindness is a term applied to children who are unable to learn to read. This defect is much more common than congenital word deafness and is more easily recognized.

While many factors play a role in reading retardation, there are some children whose reading disability is due to congenital lack of the ability to appreciate the significance of visual symbols. This is truly congenital word blindness. It can conceivably be due to incomplete development or an aplasia in the visual word area of the cortex located in the angular gyrus, Brodman's area 39. Drew (18) believes in a dominant genetic factor in some forms of dyslexia and postulates that the disability is due to failure of maturation of the parietal lobes. Kawi and Pasamanick (19) compared male children having reading disorders with a control group. They found that children with reading disabilities had a significantly larger proportion of premature births and abnormalities of the prenatal and paranatal periods than the control subjects. The toxemias and bleeding during pregnancy constituted those complications largely responsible for the differences found between the two groups.

The children with reading disabilities may exhibit right and left confusion, mixed eye and hand preference, and some motor awkwardness. These disturbed spatial orientations may have features suggesting Gerstmann's syndrome, due to involvement of the parieto-occipital regions. Gerstmann's syndrome is a complex disorder of language function due to a lesion in the angular and the supramarginal gyri. This gives rise to alexia, astereognosis, apraxia, amnesic aphasia, anomia, and hemianopia.

Orton (7) demonstrates that many children suffering from congenital word blindness exhibit mirror-writing tendencies, which may be secondary to mirror-reading ("no" is pronounced as "on"). He attributes this disorder to lack of development of cerebral dominance. Many of these children also have difficulty in spelling. Orton named this condition *strephosymbolia,* which means "twisted symbols."

One may compare word deafness in children with word blindness. Both are defects in the zone of language, but word blindness is more easily recognized and has been more frequently reported. Undoubtedly, many children with word deafness are diagnosed and treated as deaf mutes or are regarded as mentally retarded children. Congenital word deafness, like congenital word blindness, is much more common in males than in females. The proportion is approximately five to one. It is interesting to note that the same ratio is found among stutterers. Congenital word deafness and alexia are frequently familial and may appear in different members of successive generations.

Agraphia

The counterpart of motor aphasia at the visual aphasic level is congenital motor agraphia. Agraphia, or loss of the ability to write, is infrequently seen alone, since its anatomical representation encompasses a very small area near the centers that control movement of the hands and the centers for speech production. The area for writing occupies the posterior part of the second frontal gyrus. Although agraphia may coexist with reading disability and its associated difficulty in spelling, it can exist as a separate, isolated developmental disorder. In many cases of agraphia, there is a history of a shift from the left to the right hand in infancy, or a forced training of the right hand for writing in spite of a strong left sided preference.

CLINICAL PICTURE OF CHILDHOOD APHASIAS

Letters are signs for sounds. In addition, written words are symbols, for they have content and meaning. Aristotle, in *On Interpretation,* said, "Spoken words are the symbols of mental experience and written words are the symbols of spoken words."

Words also derive their meaning through a process of association. To convey an idea, one uses a series of interrelated words, so called propositional speech. An aphasic patient manifests an inability to deal with propositional speech as well as with symbols. The aphasic may have difficulty not only in expressing himself, but he may also lack comprehension of speech as well as reading and writing.

A common observation in the language disturbance of the aphasic is his inability to use words to express thoughts and ideas, although he may use them under emotional stimulation. The intellectual component of speech may be grossly affected without proportional impairment of non-intellectual speech. Thus, an aphasic can often ejaculate words emotionally which he cannot use in correct, logical speech. An aphasic patient may swear with fluency, while no amount of urging will bring forth the same words in the form of calm, logical expression of an idea. The only words that an aphasic may have left to him are *yes* and *no,* which he may repeat constantly. Furthermore, he may say *yes* when he means *no,* and realize his mistake when questioned about his answer.

Automatic Speech

An aphasic may have little difficulty with *automatic speech.* Automatic speech consists of material which is memorized in a given order since early childhood, such as familiar verses or prayers. Thus, some aphasics may be able to recite poems or sing songs, but are unable to use the very same words in meaningful speech. In the same category may be placed the aphasic's ability to reproduce series of words such as the alphabet, days of the week, or months of the year. He may not be able to tell the specific day of the week, but when asked to start with Sunday and proceed to name the days in sequence, he will immediately recognize the specific day when he comes to it in succession. This is the type of speech that has become so thoroughly organized, systematized, and automatic, that it is only faintly voluntary. This automatic, emotional, serial, non-intellectual type of speech frequently remains relatively intact with many aphasic patients. Jackson's law of evolution and dissolution of nervous function is applicable here. The more voluntary function (intellectual speech) suffers first and most severely. The automatic function (non-intellectual speech) suffers least or not at all.

Some aphasics, especially those who after a period of time

show improvement in their linguistic ability, will speak in a very deliberate manner, pausing and groping for the proper word to express their thoughts. One can almost sense the effort they use in speaking. This slower reaction time of the aphasic is in keeping with Goldstein's hypothesis that all direct damage to the cerebral cortex causes a rise of threshold and retardation of excitation. The receptivity of the patient is reduced and it takes him longer to react.

Agrammatism, Paraphasia, Perseveration

Aphasics will frequently exhibit *agrammatism*. The agrammatism of the aphasic results from an inability to recall sentence structure. The severe stutterer may also speak agrammatically. However, the stutterer's lack of correct grammar results from the conscious avoidance of words which seem difficult for him, and the lack of ability to think immediately of a suitable substitute. This disturbance has led some investigators to consider stuttering as an associative aphasia.

Some aphasics demonstrate a *telegram style* of speech in which prepositions or articles are omitted. These articles are not strictly necessary for comprehension, but are nevertheless essential for correct speaking.

Aphasics may also exhibit *paraphasia* in which the appropriate word is replaced by a less appropriate one, which still retains a certain relationship to the correct word. Paraphasia is garbled speech. Words are either so altered in construction as to make them difficult to recognize, or are used incorrectly as in the expression, "The pleasure is all yours." *Jargon aphasia* is a more severe degree of paraphasia. Although true paraphasia represents a definite organic deficiency in the cerebral mechanism for speech, it may be a purely functional phenomenon under certain circumstances. These non-organic manifestations of paraphasia may be found in conditions of fatigue, distraction, or excessive alcoholic intake. It is important to note, however, that while the organic symptoms of paraphasia are frequently of longer duration, the non-organic, functional signs of this disability are merely transient.

At times, the attention of the aphasic becomes fixed on a letter, a word, or an idea. This fixation is called *perseveration*. A tendency toward perseveration is evident not only in speech, but also in other motor performances of the brain-damaged individual.

Concerning the intellectual changes, one may say that in every impairment of speech, there is to a certain degree an impairment of psychic function. To specify where the speech defect ends and the general intellectual defect begins is obviously impossible. It can be stated, however, that the intellectual impairment of the aphasic is not as great as would appear from his language impairment. The intellectual impairment is evidenced in slower thought processes and impairment of abstract thinking. The aphasic has difficulty in dealing with the imagined. An aphasic may be unable to use the term *red* in a sentence, but is able to say *red rose* or *red dress*. He has memory defects and disturbances in concentration and attention.

The personality modification of the aphasic may be only an exaggeration of his premorbid personality traits. In general, he demonstrates ego orientation. There may be irritability, fatigability, anxiety, or euphoria. The aphasic has a reduced ability to adjust to new situations. There is a tendency to social withdrawal and shyness.

Motor and Sensory Aphasia

In motor aphasia or aphemia (Broca's aphasia), the individual knows what he wants to say, understands spoken or written language, but is unable to express himself. Usually a few words or phrases can be said. There is considerable perseveration. The utterances are not meaningful and have no propositional value. Speech may be produced under emotional stress.

In sensory aphasia (Wernicke's aphasia), the individual is unable to understand the meaning of spoken or written language. In contrast to the motor aphasic who is often speechless, the sensory aphasic is often quite talkative. Because he does not appreciate the mistakes he makes, he is not perturbed, unlike the motor aphasic who knows what he wants to say but cannot say it. Furthermore, if meaningful motor speech is retained while the understanding of language is lost, the patient's responses are usually irrelevant. Whether disturbances in the sensory cortical sphere are due to *agnosia* or aphasia is at times difficult to determine. The ability to repeat a word implies recognition but not necessarily understanding.

A peripheral hearing loss can also accompany sensory aphasia. Loss of perception and discrimination in the upper frequency range renders the child unable to perceive and initiate consonants. Loss of perception and discrimination in the middle frequency area makes the child unable to handle vowels, semi-vowels, and nasals.

In the mixed type of aphasia, both understanding and expression are lost, a general attitude of apathy results and the individual may give the impression of being deaf. It is significant that most aphasics are of the mixed type, with a preponderance of either sensory or motor involvement. Indeed, some investigators would emphatically deny the existence of a purely receptive or expressive aphasia.

In *amnesic aphasia,* the individual may recognize a word, can use it soon afterward, but after a short period is unable to reproduce it. The patient is able to talk and has a clear idea about what he wants to say, but he lacks the words. However, if he is allowed to hear or see the phrases he wants to use, he understands them at once and uses them, even through he does not retain the words in his memory constellation.

Reading aphasics (non-readers) exhibit persistent school failure in reading, writing, and spelling. An emotional overlay, frequently asocial, is an expected secondary result. The non-reader also exhibits a tendency to alter the directions of writing not only in the horizontal axis (reversals), but also in the vertical axis (inversions). In inversions, the individual makes pencil strokes from below upward. In short, reading aphasics frequently present with a double axial rotation. Mixed laterality is also noted.

The defects observed in aphasics are not always constant. The individual may be able to perform in an area that was previously faulty. However, such achievements are only transitory.

Emotional Problems

Disturbances in language function are only one aspect of childhood aphasia. These children usually present, in varying degree, behavioral changes in the intellectual and emotional field, as well as marked changes in the general personality make-up. There is a tendency toward social withdrawal, shyness, and seclusiveness, although the child usually reacts normally to those stimuli in his environment which he is able to understand. The child is, at times, aggressive and irritable without what would seem to be normal provocation. He presents easy fatigability and distractibility. On intelligence tests, he usually shows a scattered picture, being strikingly backward in verbal tests and showing normal responses in performance tests. He is usually skillful in his movements. These behavior and personality patterns may be due to the altered physiological relationships of the cortex. There is no doubt, however, that these personal traits may also be the result of a psychoneurotic reaction to an environment that is lacking in understanding. The effect of aphasia on the child is to interfere with educational progress. The more severely handicapped aphasics may not be educable through ordinary means. Some of the children, if the difficulty is unrecognized, may become "imbeciles from deprivation."

There is hardly a symptom or sign in aphasia resulting from an organic lesion that has not also been noted in purely functional states. Fright may be a cause of mutism similar to that seen in aphasia. Inability to recall names of familiar persons may be a purely functional problem as well as a primary sign of organic disease. Thus, personality disorders may either arise from organic lesions or may result from purely functional problems.

DIAGNOSIS AND DIFFERENTIAL DIAGNOSIS

It is much more difficult to make a diagnosis of childhood aphasia than adult aphasia. In childhood aphasia, there is a retardation in symbolic communication, while in adult aphasia, there is a loss, a deficit, in the use of symbols.

Concerning specific tests for the diagnosis of childhood aphasia, there is at present no generally accepted method of testing the aphasic. Adult tests for aphasia, while designed to evaluate the patient's specific language disturbances, place a great deal of stress on evaluating the patient's disabilities in perceptual, organizational, and conceptual spheres. Since young children, and especially children who have disturbances of language function, still have not fully developed higher abstract thought processes, tests used with aphasic adults have only limited value.

Each aphasic child should have a complete physical and neurological examination, including hearing and visual acuity tests. Evaluation of family history and emotional status should be made. Psychometric tests, tests for various modalities of language function and handedness determination should be given.

Because aphasia is a disorder of language, it is a distinctly human disability. The problem does not lend itself to experimental research with animals. The question is often asked about the earliest age at which an aphasic child can be detected. The answer is probably not before two and one-half years of age. That is the time when the child's speech development will lag behind expectation. That is the time when language and other intellectual abilities can be tested separately. The diagnosis of congenital aphasia is based upon symptoms. The child may require a period of study and observation of behavior patterns before the diagnosis can be made. Physical examination is usually negative. There are no specific neurological signs. Tests of postural responses, which have been reported to be abnormal in children with reading disabilities, are of no value in aphasic children under six years of age, since it is only after age six that posture becomes static enough to be of diagnostic significance. Eisenson's (20) *Examining for Aphasia* is a simple series of tests that one can use to obtain information concerning language abilities and limitations of the adolescent and adult.

Although it is common practice to arrive at a diagnosis of aphasia in children by a process of exclusion, this is not altogether necessary. Hardy (21) has outlined several procedures to help one arrive at the diagnosis.

First, one must test for auditory discrimination. This involves both pitch and loudness. Many children are thought to be aphasic whose only major problem is the incapacity to discriminate auditory stimuli.

Second, Hardy states one should study cerebral function in terms of *pattern-perception, foreground-background recognition* and the like, in both vision and audition. Many aphasic children have trouble here. One of the deficits of a highly distractible child who is not learning language, is a fundamental inability to pay consistent attention to the succession of stimuli which makes possible the learning of verbal auditory meaning. One also finds aphasic children who have as much difficulty with visual as with auditory recognition and recall. They simply cannot perform as symbolic pattern makers.

Third, one must search for basic problems of cortical integration as demonstrated in a classically aberrant electroencephalogram (EEG). For example, the characteristic changes in the EEG found in the epileptic child preclude the inclusion of this child as an aphasic, although the child is frequently aphasoid in his behavior at some stages in development.

Fourth, one must concentrate on what Hardy refers to as the status of *auditory* and *visual tracking*. Tracking is the management of sensory information in succession as a function of time and relative to the dynamics of the entire cerebrum. This kind of function has been called *serial-order temporal integration.* Tracking is a distinctly human attribute and consists of being able to process a variety of incoming information, employing all the attributes of the sensorium, and relating this information to previous and presently pertinent experiences. For example, many children at age six, achieve a six-year level in word meaning, but cannot manage the complexity of a sentence. This is a form of disability in tracking, although it is not always labeled aphasia. Hardy believes tracking is probably the most important aspect in the diagnosis of aphasia in children.

One may suspect that aphasia exists in a child under the age of two and one-half years if one observes a lack of speech development and failure of auditory or visual comprehension. However, as Wood (22) points out, the actual diagnosis of aphasia must be delayed until the child reaches the chronological age when he begins to use verbal symbols. She also states that definite diagnosis of childhood aphasia cannot be made until the child fails to perform adequately on the criterion used for diagnosis, namely, the inability to use language symbolically at a judgment level.

The striking feature about aphasics is the great disparity between language ability and the rest of the mental processes. The discrepancy between the child's lack of language development and his adequate level of hearing and normal intelligence is the key to the diagnosis. The aphasic child presents a scattered picture. He is most backward in those tests where some relation to speech exists, while he may show normal or above normal abilities in those performances which do not depend on speech.

The personality and emotional problems that many of the aphasic children present may at times be even more striking than the disturbances in language function. This often makes it difficult to make a differential diagnosis between an aphasic child and a mentally retarded, schizophrenic, or autistic child. Deafness, of course, is practically always a question with all these children. The ability to learn speech to a great extent governs the rate of development of mental capacity. Congenital deafness hinders the learning of speech and inhibits the development of normal intellectual growth.

DIFFERENTIAL DIAGNOSIS: MENTAL RETARDATION, SCHIZOPHRENIA, AUTISM VS. APHASIA

In differential diagnosis, Karlin (9) discusses each of the above mentioned disabilities in terms of developmental history, behavior, intelligence tests, speech and prognosis.

A. Mental Retardation
1. *Developmental History*: The child exhibits delay in the onset of talking, sitting, and walking.
2. *Behavior*: The child shows a limited interest in his surroundings and is easily tired. His movements are slow and awkward. The child may be placid or erethic, and if he is the latter, he may behave like a psychotic.
3. *Intelligence Tests*: There is an all-pervasive mental deficiency, although the child may present an uneven distribution of his abilities.
4. *Speech*: Language is meager and may be limited to a few irrelevant words. There is often a marked tendency toward echolalia. At best, vocabulary is scanty and there is a paucity of ideas.
5. *Prognosis*: There is some improvement with age, but basically there is not much change and the child remains on the same level.

B. Schizophrenia
1. *Developmental History*: Although there is normal onset in the ability to talk, there is lack of voluntary speech. The child exhibits normal onset of sitting and walking.
2. *Behavior*: The picture is one of lack of uniform behavior. There may be seclusiveness, immobility, and posturing. The child does not pay attention to his surroundings. His mode of thinking and acting is foreign to the life of the normal child. There is general emotional blunting or the emotional response may be out of proportion to the external situation.
3. *Intelligence Tests*: The child may be extremely backward in certain areas and surpass his own age level in others. He may be confused, even though he may possess superior intelligence.
4. *Speech*: The child may use made-up words or odd combinations of actual words. His speech may be sparse or incoherent and irrelevant.
5. *Prognosis*: Retrogression in behavior and interests becomes more marked with age.

C. Autism
1. *Developmental History*: There is a similarity between autism and schizophrenia. Although there is normal onset in the ability to talk, there is lack of voluntary speech. The child exhibits normal onset of sitting and walking.
2. *Behavior*: Withdrawal tendencies are noted early in life. There is an obsessive desire for the maintenance of sameness. Changes in routine can drive the child to despair. The child is interested in objects and plays with them, but does not pay attention to people or what they do around him. The child is happiest when left alone.
3. *Intelligence Tests*: The child resembles the schizophrenic in that he may be extremely backward in certain areas and surpass his own age level in others.
4. *Speech*: The child may remain mute. The majority, however, acquire the ability to speak. Speech, even when present, does not convey meaning to others. Nouns present no difficulty, for the child may remember long and unusual names. Delayed echolalia is present, for he may repeat at a later date a word or a sentence he heard a day or two before.
5. *Prognosis*: Little progress is made.

D. Aphasia
1. *Developmental History*: The child usually exhibits a delay in the onset of talking, although the development of sitting and walking are normal.

2. *Behavior*: There is a tendency to shyness and seclusiveness. The child reacts quite normally to those stimuli in his surroundings which he is able to understand. Due to lack of verbal comprehension, he may at times show aggressiveness and irritation.
3. *Intelligence Tests*: The child shows a scattered picture. He is strikingly backward in verbal tests, has normal responses on performance tests, and is skillful in his movements.
4. *Speech*: It may be plentiful, sparse or even absent. The child may lack comprehension or expression, depending upon whether the aphasia is sensory or motor. The child may learn to lip read or may understand gestures.
5. *Prognosis*: There is some improvement with time and adequate parental and speech therapeutic training. This will be discussed in the later sections on prognosis and treatment.

Audimutitas

Audimutitas (dumbness without deafness) must be considered in the differential diagnosis of word deafness or sensory aphasia. Audimutitas describes the condition of children who apparently are mentally normal, hear well and understand speech, but do not talk. The condition may be purely functional. The lack of speech may be due either to negativistic tendencies or due to fear reactions, as a result of environmental factors. Organic causes may also play a role. Seemann (23) points out that in children who present a pathological fetal position, audimutitas may be of cerebellar and vestibular origin. Therefore, since synergism is a fundamental cerebellar function, the evolution of speech is also contingent on an intact cerebellum.

Differential Diagnosis: Apraxia, Agnosia

Some investigators suggest that motor aphasia is a more complex form of apraxia. Apraxia, however, is the inability to perform learned, purposeful movements upon command when no motor, sensory, or intellectual impairment is present. Apraxia is an interference with the *association fibers* connecting the precentral gyrus with the higher psychic regions.

It is often very difficult to differentiate agnosia from sensory aphasia. Jackson, in 1876, called agnosia imperception. Freud, in 1891, introduced the term agnosia. If a patient understands what is said to him and has intelligible speech but cannot recognize familiar objects, then he has agnosia. If a child does not respond to speech, he may have agnosia or sensory aphasia to auditory stimuli. If he indicates that he recognizes words, but does not understand their meaning, then a sensory aphasia exists and there is no agnosia. In agnosia, speech appears like a completely strange language. In aphasia, speech sounds like a familiar language, even though it is not understood. Finally, there may be a mixture of both agnosic and aphasic symptomatology.

PROGNOSIS

Most children with aphasia can learn speech patterns. The progress in development of language in an aphasic child can be more rapid than in the adult with aphasia. Once the childhood aphasic with an organic disorder or a developmental disorder starts making progress, he can often accelerate.

The younger the age of the patient at the onset of aphasia, the better the chances for improvement, provided the child can follow a therapeutic regime. The earlier the diagnosis of aphasia is made, and the shorter the period of time between the diagnosis of aphasia and the beginning of therapy, the greater the possibility for restoration of speech. Basic to the prognosis in aphasia, however, is the severity of the original organic insult to the brain. If brain damage is mild, aphasia may be transient. If motor paralysis is widespread and severe, indicating a large lesion, then there is less likelihood for improvement to take place. In general, sensory aphasics improve to a greater degree than do motor aphasics.

A child with a higher intellectual potential can overcome handicaps better than the child with normal or low intellectual capacity. Most childhood aphasics who cannot overcome their speech disability are children whose aphasia is complicated by poor intelligence or lack of adequate hearing, and in whom school placement would have been difficult even without aphasia.

D. Karlin and Hirschenfang (24) studied the rehabilitative ability of hemiplegics with and without aphasia. It is widely believed that since right hemiplegics exhibit aphasia, they are more severely handicapped than the left hemiplegics. Left hemiplegics are considered good prospects for rehabilitation, since they have no difficulty in comprehending instructions or expressing their needs through speech. In comparing right hemiplegics with left hemiplegics, D. Karlin, and Hirschenfang found, however, that in spite of being able to communicate well, the left hemiplegics presented more visuosensory and visuomotor disturbances than did the right hemiplegics with aphasia. Therefore, the authors suggest that the right hemiplegic, even with his aphasia, offers a better chance for vocational rehabilitation than does the left hemiplegic without a speech impediment.

TREATMENT AND REHABILITATION

It is evident that in the acquired childhood aphasias resulting from encephalitis, brain abscess, or brain tumor, the paramount concern is not the treatment of the speech disability, but the treatment of the underlying condition that produces it.

The problem of aphasia, however, should be given more direct attention in those children who are either born with hemiplegia or who develop hemiplegia shortly after birth, especially if the hemiplegia is on the right side. It is true that some cases have been reported of children who were born with right hemiplegia and yet exhibited no aphasic symptoms. Krynauw (25), to relieve increased convulsive activity, removed the entire left cerebral hemisphere from a child with infantile right hemiplegia and the child learned to speak. It is assumed that speech became possible by a complete shift of function to the right hemisphere. Children of this type probably have the right arm so severely handicapped that they can make a complete shift to the left hand.

How the aphasic child regains even partial function, having had brain damage, in view of the known incapacity of the central nervous system to regenerate, is an intriguing and unsettled question. It has been suggested that there is such a phenomenon as "takeover" or regeneration of function. One theory even goes so far as to state that there is a transfer of neuronal connections and that sensory ganglion cells can become motor neurons. Another point of view contends that ipsilateral representation of speech function in the cortex is responsible for regaining activity. After examining these hypotheses, one must conclude that there is no real evidence for reorganization or "takeover" of function at any level, even in such lower forms of life as the amphibians. It is possible, however, that the reserve of potentially effective cortical tissue for a certain function is large. It is also probable that speech is a bilaterally represented function, at least in some individuals. Furthermore, in right hemiplegia, there may be an improvement in communication parallel with development of vigor in the left side of the body.

Therapeutic habilitation of the aphasic child is more effective with the less severe cases of right hemiplegia, where paresis is moderate or mild, and paralysis of the right hand is not complete. The tendency is to provide exercises for the "bad" arm and to encourage its use in an attempt to improve it. This is done, unfortunately, even to the exclusion of the "good" arm and hand. Thus, a confusion of handedness often occurs. This may delay the establishment of cerebral dominance. It might be advisable not to encourage the use of the affected side until some time after the onset of speech. Perhaps it would even be better to wait until the child is progressing normally in school. This would hasten the completion of the shift to the good arm and probably aid in the establishment of dominance.

PRINCIPLES IN THERAPY

In treating the congenitally aphasic child, Karlin (9) states that one should follow certain principles. First, there is the principle of *facilitation*. Stimulation of one neuron or an area of neurons may facilitate another area through subliminal stimulation. Thus, stimulation of one performance field may influence the performance in other parts of the same field.

Second, one should allow the aphasic child sufficiently *long exposure to the stimulus* in order to promote the greatest chance of success in a task. It has been shown that where brain damage exists, the receptivity of the patient is reduced. The reaction time is therefore prolonged.

Third, *distracting stimuli should be reduced* to a minimum during therapy, since distractibility and inability to concentrate, are common traits of aphasic children.

Fourth, *parental inclusion* must be incorporated in the treatment program. If the child exhibits word deafness, for example, the parents should try as much as possible to stimulate his interest in speech by talking to him, reading to him, and showing and describing pictures, in an effort to motivate the child's verbal communicative interests. The usual adage, "The child should be seen, not heard" should be changed to, "The child should be heard and seen." The parents should be made to understand the child's defect. They should appreciate the fact that the child has to be under observation for a long time. One must be made aware that one is dealing with a growing child and that the normal process of growth and development may produce results which no one can foretell. Therapeutic efforts should be directed to help this normal growth and development.

Finally, the most important principle in the treatment of the aphasic child is that the training in each case must involve *specific adaptation* to the individual. Basically, the emphasis should be placed on the use of unimpaired, or relatively unimpaired sensory and motor pathways, as well as on the establishment of new pathways.

The aphasic child frequently has been deluged with all kinds of verbal stimulation in his immediate surroundings, stimulation which he cannot absorb. He may even develop a resistance to the constant and persistent enticement to speak. It is perhaps better at first to reduce, rather than to concentrate the verbal stimuli.

EDUCATIONAL APPROACH

The *educational approach* includes school placement and speech therapy. Initial efforts should be directed toward socialization of the child, preferably in a kindergarten or nursery school in the company of children who speak normally. Speech skills of normal children are highest when speech is fun, when the speech situation is pleasurable and when speech contributes to the child's daily activities. Training for the aphasic must be adapted to arouse his interest and to stimulate him to use materials which he finds interesting.

At one time, it was advocated that children with sensory aphasia, namely those with auditory agnosia, be placed in a school for the deaf. While some of the methods of speech therapy used with the acoustically handicapped may be adopted in treating these children, it would be psychologically wrong to place a child with word deafness in a school for the deaf. The ideal educational situation would be a school for normal children with small classes and a teacher willing to cooperate and help the child.

SPEECH THERAPY

Speech is a moving *pattern* of sounds, in which the individual elements are disregarded. The aim, therefore, when treating aphasic children is not to build up speech sound by sound, or later word by word, but rather to build up real speech patterns. One should begin by presenting short words which are linked with an actual object or image. These words are repeated frequently. At first, one should start with nouns, then verbs and finally adjectives, adverbs and connectives. It is important to give the child encouragement and to prevent frustration.

The length of the speech therapy session depends upon the individual child's attention span. Training should involve as many sensory approaches as possible. The child should see the object or picture and should be allowed to touch it. The name should then be pronounced for him, repeated, and perhaps even written. While this is being done, it should be ascertained whether there is one approach by which the child learns more easily. This approach should then be used to fullest advantage.

Sensory (Receptive) Aphasia

Sensory or receptive aphasics are much more difficult to work with than motor or expressive aphasics, since the former do not perceive full stimuli. If an auditory agnosia is present, the patient should be encouraged to use other cues such as sight, olfactory sense, tactile and taste senses, and kinesthetic sense, to compensate for the stimuli that are blocked by the auditory disability. For example, one child could not distinguish a banana by sight or touch, but could identify it and name it when he smelled the object. After repeatedly smelling it, looking at it and handling the object, he was able to name it on sight. He admitted, however, that at times it was necessary for him to recall the smell of the fruit before he was able to give it the name "banana." Actual objects are not always necessary. Pictures of objects, miniatures, and the printed and oral word can be used as a lead-off, depending upon the patient and his potentialities.

Speech therapy is given by a trained speech clinician. Receptive aphasics who have a serious loss in the understanding of speech, should first be taught to comprehend visual cues. This may involve a simple form of lip reading, although the training may not have to be as intensive as it is with a deaf child. A hearing tube may be tried. This tube is not used as an amplifier, but rather to bring the auditory stimulus closer to the ear. By using this auditory stimulus in combination with visual symbols, auditory attention and perception are developed and trained.

The main purpose of therapy is to motivate the child's use of language in his daily activities. This is not limited to his speaking habits alone, but also involves the utilization of hearing and seeing. Children with auditory agnosia may ignore language because it is meaningless to them. In order to develop auditory word associations, the child should be encouraged to listen to spoken language as well as to rely on visual and other sensory stimulation. In cases where the audiometer test is normal, the use of a hearing aid is certainly not indicated. Furthermore, artificial methods of increasing the volume of language sound to a point beyond comfortable listening are worthless, and may be detrimental in the case where there is no hearing loss. When the level of sound is raised to the point of discomfort, the natural reaction on the part of the child will be to develop resentment toward the auditory stimulus.

Alexia and Agraphia

There are children with severe reading disabilities for whom one has to accept the diagnosis of alexia (word blindness). These are uncommon cases. At present, there are no known methods of teaching these children usable reading.

The vast majority of children with reading disabilities, however, can learn to read with special help. Most educational systems are organized on the assumption that all children are ready for initial reading instruction at about six years of age. Children differ, however, in their rate of development. Not all children are ready to read when they attain a certain chronological age. If a child who had difficulty in learning to read is promoted from grade to grade, his confusion will increase with each succeeding class, and he may develop an unfavorable attitude toward reading. Better adaptation of teaching methods for reading, to some of these deviating cases, will prevent the development of unfavorable attitudes, especially if these adaptations are made early in life. Specialists in remedial reading might well be consulted in such cases.

As for agraphia, it is practically never found by itself. Since the ability to write is dependent upon the ability to read, the child with an alexia is also unable to spell words. A further discussion of alexia and agraphia will be found in the chapter on related language disabilities.

Motor (Expressive) Aphasia

Before attempting therapy with the motor aphasic, it is necessary to know at what level the child usually performs. One must say "usually" because the motor aphasic's responses are not consistent, especially in the early stages. If the child cannot give an automatic response when asked to count from one to ten, or tell the clinician his name, this is the place to start rather than having him discuss the latest news of the day. From teaching automatic speech, it is easier to proceed to words, phrases, sentences, and finally paragraphs such as are necessary in everyday conversation. It has been found helpful to many clinicians to use more than one type of stimulus to obtain the desired result. For example, saying the numbers, writing or copying them, and reading them, can be combined for faster and more secure learning.

Other children learn best by using word couplet associations. For example, one child could only say the word "blue" when he looked at the sky and thought "blue sky." Eventually, it was not necessary to use the association. Thus, the word "blue" could be recalled without the previously used cue.

Other children with motor aphasia seem to learn faster utilizing a pencil as a crutch. They will write out the words that escape them, and then are able to read or say them. At first, the child is often encouraged to use the pencil. Some children have only to write the first letter of the word to recall it orally. Some patients can proceed from using the actual pencil to using an imaginary one on paper, or in the palm of their hand. As the child progresses, he recalls the image of the way the word is spelled and later need not use the "crutch" at all.

Often, the aphasic is given varying assignments at one time. Depending upon his level of accomplishment, he is asked to name a given set of objects, identify colors, or perform a task in daily living. As the child progresses to the point of receiving, comprehending and expressing himself more easily, he might be asked to discuss a simple story that was read to him.

Investigators have noted a relationship between the improvement of musculoskeletal function and the improvement in speech function of the motor aphasic. While this has been noted mainly in the adult aphasics with hemiplegia, it is also applicable to childhood aphasia. Tobis (26) concludes that motor experience is important for language experience. The motor act of dressing or walking may either facilitate speech or enhance the learning process that is involved in the complex system of verbal communication. According to Tobis, the patient should, therefore, be encouraged to perform muscular activities that will reinforce his language function. Thus, the physical and occupational therapists, in helping the child to improve his musculoskeletal function, are helping to improve his ability to communicate.

SUMMARY

Wood (27) has astutely made the following observation: "The apparent trend that the child with receptive aphasia becomes more like the deaf child, the child with expressive aphasia becomes more like the emotionally disturbed child and the child with mixed aphasia becomes more like the mentally retarded child as he grows older, suggests that this so-called *associative adjustment* is one type of behavioral compensation that a child may assume because of the basic aphasic condition." According to the associative adjustment theory, if the aphasia is primarily sensory, the clinician should stress the production of individual speech sounds with each sound associated with its written letter symbol. If the aphasia is primarily motor, the child responds best to whole word concepts, since he often becomes frustrated and emotionally disturbed over the production of individual sounds. Lastly, if the aphasia is both sensory and motor, therapy should utilize sound units plus whole word concepts. It should also be remembered that since the child's problems may appear different from year to year, therapy should remain quite flexible to meet the patient's variable needs.

There is a certain sequence in language development. Hearing comprehension develops ahead of propositional speech, and learning to read precedes learning to write. There is also the fact, as Karlin (28) states, that depending upon the age level of the child, the following different language disorders may present themselves in young children. Language problems become apparent at the age of two to three years if the child is aphasic. There is no speech. Between three and five years of age, during the period when the child ceases to use predominantly one word sentences and begins to express his thoughts and desires in more complex structures, some children stutter. At six or seven years of age, the problem of reading disability may present itself. All of these disorders are much more common in the male than in the female. These disabilities are frequently familial and may appear in different members of successive generations of one family tree. One must, therefore, consider the possibility of a genetically sex-linked chromosomal determinant in the genes of children exhibiting congenital aphasia, stuttering, and reading disabilities.

Karlin (28) introduces the possibility that there may be a common etiologic denominator for these language disorders. He postulates that the common etiologic factor for these disabilities may be a lack of, or delay in, maturation of certain regions in the cortex, so that the progress of a certain mode of action is deviated or inhibited. Karlin's (17) psychosomatic theory of stuttering postulating that the defect is basically an organic disorder due to a delay in myelinization of certain association areas in the brain cortex, may also find applicability to childhood aphasias and reading disabilities.

In conclusion, aphasia in children, especially congenital aphasia, is still an area where a great deal of investigation is needed. To say it does not exist is to bury one's head in the sand. Basic research in brain physiology and language function will undoubtedly shed some much needed light on this very complex, provocative, and still unsolved problem.

REFERENCES

(1a) Jackson, H.: On Affections of Speech from Disease of the Brain. *Brain, 1*:304, 1878-79.

(1b) Jackson, H.: On Affections of Speech from Disease of the Brain. *Brain, 38*:107, 1915.

(2) Goldstein, K.: *Language and Language Disturbances: Aphasic Symptom Complexes and Their Significance for Medicine and Theory of Language.* New York, Grune & Stratton, Inc., 1948.

(3) Fulton, J. F.: In, Howell, W. H.: *Textbook of Physiology.* Edited by J. F. Fulton, 17th Ed., Philadelphia, W. B. Saunders Co., 1955.

(4) Head, H.: *Aphasia and Kindred Disorders of Speech.* London, Cambridge University Press, 1926.

(5) Teitelbaum, H. A.: Analysis of Disturbances of Higher Cortical Functions, Agnosia, Apraxia, and Aphasia. *J. Nerv. & Ment. Dis.,* 97:44, January, 1943.

(6) Nielsen, J. M., and Thompson, G. N.: *The Engrammes of Psychiatry.* Springfield, Thomas, 1947.

(7) Orton, S. T.: *Reading, Writing and Speech Problems in Children: A Presentation of Certain Types of Disorders in the Development of the Language Faculty.* New York, W. W. Norton & Co., 1937.

(8) Critchley, M.: The Study of Language-Disorder: Past, Present, and Future. In, *The Centennial Lectures Commemorating the One Hundredth Anniversary of E. R. Squibb & Sons.* New York, G. P. Putnam's Sons, 1959, pp. 269-292.

(9) Karlin, I. W.: Aphasias in Children. *Am. J. Dis. Child.,* 87:752, June, 1954.

(10) Karlin, I. W.: Congenital Verbal-Auditory Agnosia (Word Deafness). *Pediatrics,* 7:60, January, 1951.

(11) Nielsen, J. M.: *Agnosia, Apraxia, Aphasia.* New York, Paul B. Hoeber, Inc., 1946.

(12) Ewing, A. W. G.: *Aphasia in Children.* London, Oxford University Press, 1940.

(13) Nance, L. S.: Differential Diagnosis of Aphasia in Children. *J. Speech Disorders, 11*:219, September, 1946.

(14) Froeschels, E.: Psychic Deafness in Children. *Arch Neurol. & Psychiat., 51*:544, June, 1944.

(15) Worster-Drought, C., and Allen, I. M.: Congenital Auditory Imperception (Congenital Word-Deafness): and its Relation to Idioglossia and Other Speech Defects. *J. Neurol. & Psychopath., 10*:193, January, 1930.

(16) Best, C. H., and Taylor, N. B.: *Physiological Basis of Medical Practice.* 7th Ed., Baltimore, Williams & Wilkins Co., 1961.

(17) Karlin, I. W.: A Psychosomatic Theory of Stuttering. *J. Speech Disorders, 12*:319, September, 1947.

(18) Drew, A. L.: A Neurological Appraisal of Familial Congenital Word-Blindness. *Brain, 79*:440, September, 1956.

(19) Kawi, A. A., and Pasamanick, B.: Association of Factors of Pregnancy with Reading Disorders in Childhood. *J. A. M. A., 166*:1420, March 22, 1958.

(20) Eisenson, J.: *Examining for Aphasia: A Manual for the Examination of Aphasia and Related Disturbances.* New York, The Psychological Corp., 1954.

(21) Hardy, W.: *Panel Discussion on Childhood Aphasia.* Palo Alto, Stanford University Institute on Childhood Aphasia, September, 1960.

(22) Wood, N.: *Panel Discussion on Childhood Aphasia.* Palo Alto, Stanford University Institute on Childhood Aphasia, September, 1960.

(23) Seemann, M.: Gehör und Sprache. *Wein. med. Wchnschr., 80*:1131, August 23, 1930.

(24) Karlin, D. B., and Hirschenfang, S.: A Comparison of Visuosensory and Visuomotor Disturbances in Right and Left Hemiplegics. *Am. J. Ophth., 50*:627, October, 1960.

(25) Krynauw, R. A.: Infantile Hemiplegia Treated by Removal of One Cerebral Hemisphere. *South African M. J., 24*:539, July 8, 1950.

(26) Tobis, J. S.: Physical Medicine and Rehabilitation Management in Aphasia. *J. A. M. A., 171*:393, September 26, 1959.

(27) Wood, N.: Personal Communication to the Authors.
(28) Karlin, I. W.: *Panel Discussion on Childhood Aphasia*. Palo Alto, Stanford University Institute on Childhood Aphasia, September, 1960.

Chapter 10

MENTAL RETARDATION

Semantics plays a great role in one's life. Parents of mentally retarded children are much happier when told that their child is "brain injured" rather than mentally retarded. The term "brain injured child" was originally restricted to children with minimal brain damage and normal family constellation. Some investigators now include in this group children with gross neurological deficits such as cerebral palsied children. It is possible, on the other hand, for a mentally retarded child to have a completely negative physical and neurological examination, and a cerebral palsied child to be normal mentally. Yet, in a sense, both these children are brain injured. The authors feel that the term "brain injured" does not denote a very precise condition. All it implies is that the pathology resides somewhere in the brain. In this chapter the attempt will be made to separate from the all-inclusive group of "brain injured" children those that specifically exhibit mental retardation.

Mental retardation may be defined as inadequate mental development which results in incapacity for independent social adaptation. Intellectual deficiency is therefore a social as well as a biological problem.

One must emphasize that the term mental retardation or mental deficiency covers a wide range between the near normal and the extremely abnormal. Three attributes are recognized in the mentally retarded. First, there is developmental or constitutional arrest. Second, intellectual retardation is present. Third, social and occupational inadequacy are evident. In some cases, favorable personality and social habits may, for a time, change marginal failure into marginal success.

An increased birth rate, a decrease in infant mortality, and a longer life span resulting from medical advances have caused a rise in the total number of persons who are mentally retarded.

RELATIONSHIP OF SPEECH TO MENTAL RETARDATION

Speech is one of the criteria often employed as an index of mental development of the child. The intellectually normal growing child not only makes sounds, but gradually associates many of these sounds with certain people and objects in his environment. Thus, sounds are progressively put together to form words and sentences used to convey meaning to others. West (1) states that language must utilize intellectual factors, since language is a process of concept building.

There is a relationship between the degree of language development and intelligence. Language deficiency has been recognized for a long time as a characteristic sign of the mentally retarded. As early as 1914, Binet and Simon (2) employed the frequent absence of language and speech in the severely mentally retarded as the basis for their definition of an "idiot." Tredgold (3) observes that in idiocy, speech is commonly absent although a few children learn monosyllabic words such as *dog, cat,* and *rat.* In no case, however, does Tredgold feel that the idiot can form sentences.

It is frequently assumed that the degree of the speech defect is directly proportional to the degree of mental retardation. Tredgold (3) points out that this premise led Esquirol to suggest that the level of speech development might be employed as a basis for classification of the mentally retarded. There are many exceptions, however, to this assumption. Some severely retarded children who have limited speech, have relatively good articulation. Other children in a higher I. Q. group may have a larger vocabulary but have many articulatory defects. In the final analysis, the severity of a child's mental retardation must not be judged solely by the degree of intelligibility or by the amount of verbalization.

In a study of the causes of delayed speech development, Karlin and Kennedy (4) state that mental retardation must be considered a possible cause when a child of two or two-and-one-half years of age shows no attempt at verbal expression. Seth and Guthrie (5) quote Mead as saying that in a study of feeble-minded individuals, the average age for inception of speech is thirty-four months, although there is a wide individual variability. Tredgold (3) states that lack of speech at the age of four years is of particular significance in the diagnosis of mental retardation. West (1) states that mutism, complete lack of speech, can be ascribed to amentia only when the amentia is on the level of the low grade idiot.

CLASSIFICATION

Mental retardation is a symptom complex rather than a disease. There exists wide variation in the severity of mental retardation. Although classifications differ considerably, the authors are of the opinion that the two criteria of *grade* and *etiology* are of prime importance. Grade refers to the degree of severity of mental retardation. Etiology refers to the cause of amentia. It may be divided into *primary* and *secondary*. The term primary refers to hereditary, endogenous mental deficiency. The term secondary refers to acquired forms resulting from a non-hereditary cause.

GRADE

Classification differs among authorities concerning terminology employed for the grade of mental deficiency. The following terminology is in general usage among many investigators in the field of mental retardation. It embraces the terms *moron, imbecile,* and *idiot.*

The term *moron* refers to the highest grade of intelligence of children exhibiting retardation. It is widely accepted in referring to individuals whose deficiency, as measured by the intelligence quotient, is in the neighborhood of fifty to seventy. It is the mildest form of mental handicap. The moron is only slightly less intelligent than the person who is considered low-normal. The moron can perform tasks that appear too monotonous to the normal person. He can, therefore, support himself in an occupation that does not require mental ability. Special classes are required for the education of this type of mentally retarded child.

The term *imbecile* refers to children in the I. Q. range of twenty-five to fifty. This grade of mentally handicapped youngster is trainable. He may be taught to take care of his own needs, but he cannot perform any tasks that could be used in gainful occupation. He may be able to take care of himself in his own home, but he cannot become self-supporting.

The most severely retarded child is termed an *idiot*, one whose intelligence quotient places him in the I. Q. range below twenty-five. Children in this group are not trainable. They require constant care all their lives. This type of child is often institution-alized.

ETIOLOGY

The etiologic factors contributing toward mental retardation are myriad. Needless to say, they form a subject beyond the scope of this book. Although many of the causative agents in mental deficiency produce abnormalities of cerebration alone, the great majority are responsible for physical as well as mental aberrations. The four etiologic factors to be discussed include: *temporal lobe epilepsy, mongolism, severe hypothyroidism (cretinism)*, and *encephalitis*.

Epilepsy

Cecil and Loeb (6) state that, "Impaired mentality, when it occurs, is the most distressing aspect of epilepsy. Fortunately, contrary to common lay and medical opinion, serious deterior-ation is unusual." In a study of the speech problems found in temporal lobe epilepsy, Bingley (7) states that *speech automatism* and *ictal aphasia* are quite frequent. Typical symptoms of sensory aphasia are also found. The prevalence of speech automatism associated with epileptic seizures has been known for quite some time. Magnus, Penfield, and Jasper (8) found it present in five out of their thirty-four cases of masticatory seizures.

Bingley (7) states that there is a close relationship between ictal aphasia and handedness. He found that in right-handed people, the close relationship between ictal aphasia and a lesion in the left cerebral hemisphere is as equally evident as that found in post-operative aphasia. However, Bingley (7) has also shown that automatic speech is not as closely related to the dominant hemisphere as are the aphasic symptoms. "In contrast to aphasic symptoms, automatic speech may be produced by discharging lesions in either lobe, possibly even more so by lesions in the recessive hemisphere." In studying the possible association between ictal aphasia and ictal speech automatism, one may say that the mechanisms for these two entities are probably independent of each other.

An analysis of the speech defects of the child with epilepsy shows that he frequently speaks slowly and in an infantile manner. Berry and Eisenson (9) state that following an attack, the child may exhibit signs of perseveration not only in his behavior, but in his speech as well. At times, the repetition of sounds and words may resemble clonic stuttering. In some epileptics having mental retardation, the lowered intelligence produces less care in articulation, with the result that the voice is often muffled and monotonous.

Mongolism

In this condition, the physical symptoms are not progressive and mentality remains stationary. The majority of these children are imbeciles or idiots and have an I.Q. range between fifteen and forty, with the upper limit in the fifties.

The speech and language disorders found in mongolism are best summarized by West, Ansberry, and Carr (1). The speech problems arise as a result of the mental retardation coupled with the musculoskeletal abnormalities. Some of the skeletal and muscular defects of mongolism that have an adverse effect on speech production are cleft lip, cleft palate, irregular shape of the tongue and mouth, and faulty dentition. Since the mongol is not intelligent enough to make a sincere effort to overcome his deficiencies, his speech impediments are more severe than similar handicaps imposed upon the child possessing a normal intellect. Since the muscles of the mongol are flabby and hypotonic, articulation is thick and clumsy and may be characterized by the term *dysarthric*. Consonants formed by the tip of the tongue are grossly defective. The hypotonia involves the laryngeal musculature with the result that the voice is hoarse and monotonous, without modulation of pitch or intensity.

Many children exhibiting mongolism have a hearing loss from nerve deafness. Furthermore, West (1) states that, "Were it not for the fact of his low intellectual level, one could describe the mongol's failures in understanding speech as aphasic. They are clearly linguistic in significance and stem from his basic associative deficiency in the area of hearing."

The mongoloid child often has a speech defect that resembles stuttering. Gottsleben (10) finds the incidence of stuttering in a group of mongoloids to be much higher than among normal children. West (1) implies that this tendency for speech blockage is not true stuttering since the mongoloid child is not embarrassed by it, and since it does not show remissions and exacerbations correlated with emotional disturbances.

Finally, since the mongoloid's social intercourse among other children is primitive and simple due to a paucity of intellectual endowment, he does not demonstrate any speech dysfunction due to psychoneuroses.

Cretinism

When severe hypothroidism develops during fetal life or in early infancy, mental retardation and dwarfism result. The mental deficiency varies from complete helplessness to moron levels. Not only the presence of mental deterioration, but delayed dentition and the occurrence of a large and fissured tongue contribute toward faulty speech.

In early infancy, one can detect a hoarseness to the cry. There is developmental delay in talking as well as in sitting up and walking.

Berry and Eisenson (9) describe the speech of the cretin as showing a delay in both linguistic and articulatory aspects. They point to the voice of the cretin as hoarse and "froglike." "In respect to articulation, a general thickness and lack of precision prevail. Errors in consonant production are almost invariable. Sound substitution, repetition of sounds, and sound omissions may be noted. Lacking good muscle tone, inclined to be easily fatigued, and deficient in ability to execute fine and precisely coordinated motor movements, neither the articulation nor the voice of the cretin can be produced efficiently."

Encephalitis

Since encephalitis is a general term referring to an inflammation of the brain, one can see that multiple speech defects may arise, depending upon what vital function has been subjected to injury. Mental deficiency frequently occurs in the post-encephalitic stage, resulting in a paucity of speech and language development. Naturally, the younger the child at the time of the brain insult, the greater the speech impediment. Since speech abnormalities are frequently associated with motor deficiencies, the child may have difficulty in expressing himself. Gerstmann and Schilder (11) note that shortly following the onset of acute encephalitis, the speech symptoms resemble stuttering. They observe that the speech is arhythmic and punctuated by blocks and tension in the speech musculature. They state that these symptoms usually disappear following the acute episode.

ABNORMALITIES IN GROWTH AND DEVELOPMENT

Children with mental retardation frequently present an all-pervasive deficiency. Many of the children, however, exhibit uneven distribution of their intellectual and performance abilities. Karlin and Strazzulla (12) find that the most pronounced deficiencies are poor reasoning, an inability to make associations and a marked inadequacy in processes that require abstraction and symbolization. These children perform better in situations with concrete materials and activities.

The disparity in the type of cortical functioning may be detected in the early growth and development of the mentally retarded. Normally the average onset for sitting is from six to eight months, walking twelve to eighteen months, and talking eighteen to nineteen months. In Table V, Karlin and Strazzulla (12) show the onset in months of sitting, walking, and talking in relation to the intelligence quotients of fifty mentally retarded children studied by them.

An examination of Table V shows that the lower the I.Q., the later the onset of sitting, walking, and talking. Furthermore, there is a comparatively greater delay in the onset of the higher levels of symbolic activities, such as speech, than in the onset of

TABLE V

Activity	Intelligence Quotient		
	15-25	*26-50*	*51-70*
Sitting	14.7	11.2	10.6
Walking	31.0	23.5	14.4
Babbling	25.0	20.4	20.8
Words	54.3	43.2	34.5
Sentences	153.0	93.0	89.4

Table V. Age in months of the onset of certain activities in relation to intelligence quotients. From Isaac W. Karlin and Millicent Strazzulla's Speech and Language Problems of Mentally Deficient Children, *The Journal of Speech and Hearing Disorders*, 17:286, 1952. Courtesy of American Speech and Hearing Association, Washington, D. C.

the predominantly motor activities of sitting and walking. Karlin and Strazzulla also point out that in comparison with the normal, mentally retarded children exhibit a greater lag between the onset of words and the onset of simple sentences. Karlin postulates that regardless of the final intellectual endowment of the mentally deficient child, his maturation process proceeds at a much slower rate than that of the normal. This is especially pronounced in areas that are concerned with higher intellectual functions.

Criteria for intellectual levels and indices of speech acquisition are not uniform among investigators. Earlier studies by Lapage (13), Mead (14), and Wallin (15), however, support Karlin's work (see Table VI). This shows that the mentally retarded child acquires speech and language considerably later than the child of normal intelligence.

LATERALITY AND INTELLIGENCE QUOTIENT

An important feature of the human brain is the dominance of one cerebral hemisphere over the other in the performance of language function. Cerebral dominance is related to laterality, and especially to handedness, since in the right handed child the cerebral speech areas are situated in the left or dominant hemisphere.

TABLE VI

SUMMARY OF STUDIES ON USE OF FIRST WORD BY MENTALLY RETARDED

Investigator	Type Population	Time of Use of First Word	
Karlin & Strazzulla (1952)	I.Q.'s from 15-20	54	months
Karlin & Strazzulla (1952)	I.Q.'s from 26-30	43.2	months
Lapage (1911)	Low-grade defectives	41	months
Karlin & Strazzulla (1952)	I.Q.'s from 51-70	34.5	months
Mead (1913)	Nondefined retarded population	34.44	months
Wallin (1949)	Morons	18	months

Table VI. Summary of studies on use of first word by mentally retarded. From J. E. Wallace Wallin's *Children with Mental and Physical Handicaps*, 1949. Courtesy of Prentice-Hall, Inc., Englewood Cliffs, New Jersey.

Nielsen (16) states that the body scheme is related to handedness and language. It is on the basis of handedness and language that the major and minor sides are differentiated. Goldstein (17) observes that the development of cerebral dominance seems to parallel the development of higher mental functions. Differentiation in the use of the hands begins at the same time. Gesell (18) notes that a consistent laterality in both handedness and footedness shows itself in all children. McCarthy (19) states that lateral dominance apparently becomes established toward the end of the first year of life and during the first months of the second year, which is just the period when speech begins to emerge from the infant's early babbling.

Karlin (12) states that, "It would appear that there is a close interdependence between the development of cerebral dominance, laterality (especially handedness), and language function. One may postulate that the dominance of one cerebral hemisphere is the primary condition which influences the development of laterality. It is also possible that laterality, a morphological phenomenon, results in the preference of one side of the body, usually the right side. This causes a richer flow of sensory impulses to the opposite cerebral hemisphere and is a factor in establishing cerebral dominance. The question of which one comes first cannot be answered at present, and at any rate, would be purely an academic question. The best that can be said is that cerebral dominance, language function, and handedness are processes that are interrelated and no doubt influence one another developmentally."

In correlating handedness with mental retardation, Goldstein (17) observes that differentiation in the use of the hands is delayed or absent in mental deficiency. Wile (20) states that a high per cent of left handedness is frequent among children with amentia. Gordon (21) reports 18.2 per cent of mentally retarded children to be left handed while only 7.3 per cent of normal children exhibit preference for the left hand. Karlin and Strazzulla (12) studied the relationship between handedness and intelligence in mentally defective children. Table VII shows the per cent of children in whom handedness is established in relation to the intelligence quotient. It is statistically significant that as the level of the group I.Q. increases, the greater is the per cent of established handedness.

TABLE VII

I. Q. Range	C. A.°	M. A.†	Handedness Established
15-25	3 yr. 9 mo. to 14 yr. 0 mo.	0 yr. 6 mo. to 3 yr. 9 mo.	56%
26-50	3 yr. 0 mo. to 13 yr. 7 mo.	1 yr. 3 mo. to 6 yr. 0 mo.	65%
51-70	3 yr. 9 mo. to 14 yr. 1 mo.	1 yr. 8 mo. to 7 yr. 11 mo.	92%

°Chronological Age
†Mental Age

Table VII. Per cent of children in whom handedness is established in relation to intelligence quotient. From Isaac W. Karlin and Millicent Strazzulla's Speech and Language Problems of Mentally Deficient Children, *The Journal of Speech and Hearing Disorders*, 17:286, 1952. Courtesy of American Speech and Hearing Association, Washington, D. C.

SPEECH DEFECTS

There are two characteristic signs in the speech development of the mentally retarded. First, speech is frequently delayed.

Second, when speech finally does emerge, it is often defective.

Some authorities state that the speech abnormalities of the mentally deficient differ from the speech problems found in non-retarded children. Irwin (22) believes that the retarded child is not only delayed in speech production, but that his entire course in the development of sounds differs from that found in normal children. He finds that mentally retarded children use front vowels more frequently than back vowels. Their speech, therefore, resembles that of the infant more than that of the adult. Retarded children show concentration in the labial, post-dental, and glottal sounds.

Karlin, Youtz, and Kennedy (23), in a study of speech defects in young children, state that the majority of the mentally retarded have speech disorders that are similar to those of the child possessing average normal intelligence, but that the defects are more numerous and more severe in the retarded group. Matthews (24) also believes that speech defects in the mentally retarded are similar in kind to those found in a nonmentally retarded population of speech defectives.

The most common speech defects of the mentally retarded consist of *articulatory disorders, stuttering, voice problems,* and speech difficulties due to *hearing loss.*

Articulatory Defects

Karlin and Strazzulla (12) studied the frequency of consonant dysfunction in the mentally retarded. They found the most common defects to be *omission* and *substitution of sounds.* Table VIII lists the frequency of consonant defects in order of occurrence. The most frequently occurring defective consonant was *s.* It is evident from Table VIII that lisping is prevalent among these children. It is also noteworthy that Karlin finds the chief difficulties are with consonants rather than with vowels. Matthews (24) states that Karlin's findings are similar to the order of occurrence of articulatory errors that others have found in the nonretarded population.

Karlin finds that some children in the lowest I.Q. range have better articulation of sounds than children with higher I.Q.s up to seventy. Although no factual basis has as yet been given to

TABLE VIII

Sound	No. of Cases	Sound	No. of Cases
s	25	t	11
z	24	d	11
l	23	j	10
r	19	ŋ	10
tʃ	16	p	9
dʒ	16	ʒ	7
ð	16	f	6
ʃ	15	m	6
θ	15	h	6
g	14	n	5
k	14	b	3
v	12	w	3

Table VIII. Frequency of consonant defects in order of occurrence. From Isaac W. Karlin and Millicent Strazzulla's Speech and Language Problems of Mentally Deficient Children, *The Journal of Speech and Hearing Disorders, 17*:286, 1952. Courtesy of American Speech and Hearing Association, Washington, D. C.

account for this occurrence, Karlin offers two possible explanations. First, since children of the lowest I.Q. level have a very limited vocabulary, the chances for articulatory defects to develop are lessened. Second, since echolalia is more pronounced in this group, these children may be more capable of repeating a sound as they hear it.

Stuttering

Statistics differ as to whether there is a higher incidence of stuttering in the mentally retarded child. Karlin (25) found approximately the same two per cent incidence of stuttering in his work with mental defectives as he did in the normal school population.

If one takes the specific entity of mongolism, however, one finds reports to indicate that this form of mental retardation carries with it a higher incidence of stuttering than is found in the normal childhood population. Gottsleben (10) shows a thirty-three per cent incidence of stuttering in mongoloids as contrasted to an incidence of fourteen per cent in a control group consisting of nonmongoloid mental defectives. The high incidence of stuttering found in mongoloids by Gottsleben is consistent with observations made by Travis (26) and Gens (27).

Voice Problems

The chief difficulties with voice production observed by Karlin and Strazzulla (12) are nasality and huskiness, with the latter predominant among mongoloid children. Since retardates frequently have defects in their musculoskeletal systems, one can easily see how these congenital anomalies can affect many of the organs of speech. Thus, as has already been mentioned, the hypotonia of the laryngeal musculature found in the mongoloid child results in a hoarse and monotonous voice. Similarly, the presence of cleft palate produces the well known nasal quality to the voice.

Hearing Defects

The presence of auditory defects is common in many children exhibiting mental retardation. The loss of adequate hearing acuity is responsible for many speech and voice defects. Although the incidence of hearing loss in the mentally retarded differs with many authorities, most investigators believe that the per cent of hearing loss is far greater than that found in the non-retarded population.

DEFECTS IN LANGUAGE DEVELOPMENT

Defects in language function and development are as important in the mentally retarded child as the disorders of speech just enumerated. One finds great individual variability in the language ability of children with mental handicaps. Karlin and Strazzulla (12) find that some children can conduct a simple conversation with their limited vocabulary, while others of approximately the same age and intelligence, are able to say only a few meaningless words. By and large, however, children with higher mental endowment possess better language ability.

Karlin observes that a striking characteristic shown by the majority of mentally retarded children is their use of concrete language. Best responses are given in terms of objects with which the child is familiar, as in naming a pen and telling its use. Many mentally retarded children, especially those with low intelligence quotients, exhibit a marked tendency toward echolalia, repeating a question as it was given to them instead of answering it. The questions are usually repeated with the same inflection and accompanied by the same facial expression and movement as used by the interrogator.

Mentally deficient children show a paucity of ideas, lack of abstract thinking and irrelevancy of ideas. Frequently, words and sentences are introduced haphazardly with no relation to the subject matter of the conversation. There is a tendency toward perseveration.

In addition to the lack of abstract thinking, irrelevancy of ideas, echolalia, and a tendency to perseverate, Karlin and Strazzulla (12) observe that many mentally retarded children show poor attention span, accompanied by easy fatigability and distractibility. To a great extent, these symptoms resemble the symptom complex seen in aphasia. The difference, however, becomes apparent when one examines the underlying mechanism. Karlin states that many times, "In aphasia, a previously normal individual has sustained brain damage, and the deterioration in language function is one of the outstanding signs. In the mentally deficient child, the outstanding feature is the *all-pervasive* lack of development of the intellectual functions of the brain and the language defect is a secondary symptom."

It is interesting to note that Marie (28) attributed all aphasic phenomena to intellectual deficiency, an assertion which, as Wechsler (29) says, is only relatively true. Karlin and Strazzulla (12) have observed some mentally retarded children, however, whose lack of language function is out of proportion to their general intellectual retardation. They show the symptoms one sees in aphasia to such a marked degree that one is tempted to make the diagnosis of aphasia. The term aphasic, if used in these cases, should simply denote the defect in language function as the outstanding symptom and out of proportion to the general retardation of the child.

DIAGNOSIS

The question of whether a delay or a disorder in speech development can be attributed to mental retardation is, at times, difficult to answer. Certainly, if intellectual retardation is discovered, as exhibited by an intelligence quotient below seventy, mental retardation must play a part in the process.

Endocrine dysfunction, brain injury, hearing loss, and emotional disturbances can all produce deficiencies in the development of language, or result in poor articulation of sounds. If intellectual retardation does not form a part of the symptom complex, then mental retardation must be discarded as the etiologic factor responsible for the poor speech.

Aphasia, agnosia, and apraxia have all been described in the mentally retarded child. The factor of mental retardation should be considered in these cases of language dysfunction, even though the primary problem may appear to be aphasia, hearing loss, or emotional disturbance. The differential diagnosis of all these entities has already been discussed in the chapter on aphasia. One should not forget that a child labeled as aphasic or psychotic may also be mentally retarded.

TREATMENT

In order to develop normal speech and hearing, the child must have a normal central nervous system, normal intellectual endowment, adequate hearing, and stimulating social intercourse in the environment. Although all four factors may play a part in the speech disorders of the mentally retarded, the lack of adequate cerebral function is the basis for the inadequacies in speech and language communication. Psychological factors also play a part in the dysfunction of speech found in a retardate, perhaps even more than in the child possessing normal intelligence.

During the early formative years, retarded children live in a very sheltered, protective, and tense environment. Many parents have difficulty in developing a positive attitude toward the solution of the problems of the mentally deficient child. There is frequently the thought in the parents' mind, "What does the future hold for my child?" Not only do the parents have to adjust themselves to the reality of accepting the child as he is, but they also have to adjust themselves socially.

Karlin (12) states that possibly as a result of guilt feelings or overprotection, the parents develop an intense loyalty to the child and isolate him from the social life of the community. The mother constantly watches, guards, and tries to do everything for the child. This prevents the development of functions which the child can perform, given the opportunity. To protect her ego and to avoid possible remarks from the neighbors, the mother may not allow her child to play with younger children. Many parents are unable to accept their child's retardation and, as he grows older, demand educational achievements which the child is unable to attain. Since speech development is delayed, predominantly non-verbal communication such as gestures, instead of verbal relationships, are often established between child and mother. This tendency continues even when the child begins to talk, so that motivation for language development is blunted. As a result of the complex picture that the mentally retarded child presents, speech therapy must become a teamwork project interrelating the medical, psychological, social, and educational aspects of the problem.

Language and Speech Therapy

Actual speech therapy should not concern itself initially with the correction of defective sounds, but with the motivation and utilization of language. Any effort that the child makes toward communication should be encouraged even if his meaning is not clear or if he does not express himself well. If the child is mute, he should be encouraged to babble and his babblings should be repeated so that the child develops an awareness, interest, and need for speech. The child should be taught to imitate noises of cars, airplanes, and animals as part of becoming aware of sounds. Concepts must be presented to him in familiar, concrete form. His everyday surroundings should be broken down into simple units. For example, a toy house should be used and divided into as many units as there are rooms in his own home. If a doll's house is not available, a series of pictures representing various rooms may be used. A game may be played, naming the furnishings and correlating them with their use. This is followed by simple conversation centering around the rooms and their contents. The same principle may be followed with food, clothing, and other essentials in everyday living.

Various methods must be devised to encourage attention span. Clay modeling, drawing, bead stringing, block building, and other activities may be used. Since relationships with people and objects are often faulty, and since visuomotor coordination is often lacking, these methods will help strengthen these functions and consequently aid in the motivation of oral comprehension and communication.

Motivation in the use of oral language is a necessary prerequisite for any speech training. A multisensory approach should be utilized in teaching speech and language. The child should hear the word, feel the resonance of the larynx, nose, and lips, and should receive help through jaw manipulation. One technique found to be useful is to use a doll or a puppet for instruction. The child becomes the doll's speech teacher for the purpose of "instructing it to talk." All suggestions or corrections are addressed to the doll. In this manner, it has been found that the child does not feel penalized or corrected himself. During some of the sessions, the parents are encouraged to sit in on this activity, and are asked to continue the program at home. They are further advised not to anticipate the child's wishes so that he will have to use some verbal sounds to express his needs.

While the child's language progress is usually dependent upon his mental age, he may, with proper training, be able to acquire some simple abstract concepts. He may begin to distinguish colors and name them correctly, or he may use the over-all word "animals" when viewing a picture of a group of various farm animals. Karlin (12) believes that corrective speech therapy of distorted or omitted sounds should be introduced gradually, following the same principles as are used with normal children. In cases where handedness has not been developed, it is advisable to encourage the establishment of handedness by regularly instructing the child in the use of one hand in daily activities.

Educational Approach

There are special classes for the mentally retarded in most public school systems. These classes are arranged as follows: First, those who have an I.Q. of fifty to seventy are considered *educable* and are given suitable curricula and specially trained teachers. Second, those with an I.Q. of twenty to fifty are considered *trainable* and are given suitable materials and training by special teachers. In some public schools, both these groups receive training in speech and language.

Freeman and Lukens (30) describe a program in a school district in the state of Michigan. The authors feel that often these children use language that is limited even far beyond that to be expected from the extent of their mental retardation. In their program speech specialists examine every child in classes for the mentally retarded, diagnose his speech problem, and plan and direct a program formed to improve skills in verbal communication. The speech clinician also treats those children who have speech or language difficulties "unattributable to depressed intellectual function." As a result of the report of Freeman and Lukens, special teachers of the mentally retarded are forming a curriculum for oral communication in the public school system.

In the City of New York, a speech curriculum bulletin (31) has been issued and is being used in from 700 to 800 classes for mentally retarded children. This bulletin provides for two approaches to the teaching of speech skills to the retarded. One approach is through the direct teaching of the sounds of English to improve articulation and, therefore, intelligibility. The second approach is through the speech arts of story telling and reporting, choral speaking, role playing, and puppetry. The bulletin also provides for lessons in listening, auditory training in discrimination, and exercises in articulation and relaxation. The goals of this program in speech for the retarded are: first, expansion of language range in both comprehension and production; second, the improvement of speech to provide higher intelligibility in utterance. According to classroom teachers of the mentally deficient, the direct teaching of the sounds of English and how they are made, is more effective than relying on imitation alone or simply talking about the sounds.

SPECIFIC ETIOLOGIC THERAPY

The treatment of the speech and language defects in *epilepsy, mongolism, cretinism,* and *encephalitis* vary considerably. Drugs to combat the fundamental cause (the convulsions in epilepsy, the hypothyroid state in cretinism, and the acute infection in encephalitis) form the basic part of the physician's therapy. As far as mongolism is concerned, since the etiology remains unknown, no definite drug therapy can be instituted for the basic deficiencies.

Epilepsy

Infantilism is one of the problems encountered in epilepsy. A speech training program should be devised to include procedures attempting to overcome this tendency toward immature behavior.

Mongolism

West (1) states that, "The true mongol is particularly unresponsive to speech rehabilitation and it is practically useless to attempt such training." Speech therapy is usually not given to the mongol with an intelligence quotient in the idiot range, since there is no capacity to learn in this group. However, although the most severely mentally retarded are extremely difficult to rehabilitate as far as speech is concerned, some investigators believe that the child's handicap can be lessend by attempting to improve articulation.

Cretinism

Berry and Eisenson (9) believe that unless endocrine therapy shows results and the rate of maturation and development is accelerated, speech therapy is likely to be wasted on the cretin. They state that if, with endocrine treatment, physical and mental improvement is noted, a speech program should be instituted. Berry and Eisenson feel that speech improvement is often very rapid when accompanied by thyroid therapy. These authors believe that little time need be spent with voice improvement.

With improved muscular tone coupled with an awareness of the significance of speech, they feel that the voice will show considerable improvement.

Encephalitis

Investigators agree that all attempts at speech therapy for children with encephalitis should be deferred until the acute process has resolved. Once this has taken place, speech therapy can be instituted. It frequently consists of methods to improve the child's motor functions.

SUMMARY

The pediatrician often performs the first evaluation which leads parents to recognize that what appears to be a speech problem is actually a more basic problem of mental retardation. In working with all these children, parents and therapists must realize that the aim is not to attain perfect speech, but to assist the child in developing *usable,* everyday language to the maximum of his ability. One should learn to accept and strive for language and speech appropriate to mental age rather than to chronological age. Group activities can be profitably employed. The final results will depend upon the child's innate potentialities, the cooperation from the home environment, and the educational and social facilities available in the community.

REFERENCES

(1) West, R., Ansberry, M., and Carr, A.: *The Rehabilitation of Speech.* New York, Harper & Brothers, 1957.

(2) Binet, A., and Simon, T.: *Mentally Defective Children.* London, Edward Arnold, 1914.

(3) Tredgold, A. L.: *A Textbook of Mental Deficiency.* Baltimore, Williams & Wilkins Co., 1947.

(4) Karlin, I. W., and Kennedy, L.: Delay in the Development of Speech. *Am. J. Dis. Child., 51:*1138, 1936.

(5) Seth, G., and Guthrie, D.: *Speech in Childhood.* London, Oxford University Press, 1935.

(6) Cecil, R. L., and Loeb, R. F.: *A Textbook of Medicine.* Philadelphia, W. B. Saunders Co., 1963.

(7) Bingley, T.: Mental Symptoms in Temporal Lobe Epilepsy and Temporal Lobe Gliomas. *Acta Psychiatrica et Neurologica Supplementum, 120,* 33 Kobenhavn, Ejnar Munksgaard, 1958.

(8) Magnus, O., Penfield, W., and Jasper, H.: Mastication and Consciousness in Epileptic Seizures. *Acta Psychiat. et Neurol., 27*:91, 1952.

(9) Berry, M. F., and Eisenson, J.: *The Defective in Speech.* New York, F. S. Crofts & Co., 1942.

(10) Gottsleben, R. H.: The Incidence of Stuttering in a Group of Mongoloids. *Train. Sch. Bull., 62*:209, 1955.

(11) Gerstmann, J., and Schilder, P.: Studien über Bewungstörungen, über die Typen Extrapyramidaler Sprannungen und über die Extrapyramidal pseudobulbarparalyse (Akinetischhypotonisches Bulbar Syndrom). *Zeitschrift Für Die Gasamte Neurologie und Psychiatrie,* 68-70, 35-54, 1921.

(12) Karlin, I. W., and Strazzulla, M.: Speech and Language Problems of Mentally Deficient Children. *J. Speech & Hearing Disorders, 17*:286, 1952.

(13) Lapage, C. P.: *Feeblemindedness in Children of School Age.* Manchester, University Press, 1911.

(14) Mead, C. D.: The Age of Walking and Talking in Relation to General Intelligence. *Pedagogical Seminary, 20*:461, 1913.

(15) Wallin, J. E. W.: *Children with Mental and Physical Handicaps.* New York, Prentice-Hall, 1949.

(16) Nielsen, J. M.: *Agnosia, Apraxia, Aphasia.* New York, Paul B. Hoeber, 1946.

(17) Goldstein, K.: *Language and Language Disturbances.* New York, Grune & Stratton, 1948.

(18) Gesell, A.: The Ontogenesis of Infant Behavior. In, Carmichael, L.: *Manual of Child Psychology.* New York, John Wiley, 1954.

(19) McCarthy, D.: Language Development in Children. In, Carmichael, L.: *Manual of Child Psychology.* New York, John Wiley, 1954.

(20) Wile, I. S.: *Handedness Right and Left.* Boston, Lothrop, Lee, and Shepard, 1934.

(21) Gordon, H.: Left Handedness and Mirror Writing Especially Among Defective Children. *Brain, 43*:313, 1921.

(22) Irwin, O. C.: The Developmental Status of Speech Sounds of Ten Feebleminded Children. *Child. Develop., 13*:29, 1942.

(23) Karlin, I. W., Youtz, A. C., and Kennedy, L.: Distorted Speech in Young Children. *Am. J. Dis. Child.*, 59:1203, 1940.

(24) Matthews, J.: Speech Problems of the Mentally Retarded. In, Travis, L. E.: *Handbook of Speech Pathology*. New York, Appleton-Century-Crofts, 1957.

(25) Karlin, I. W.: Stuttering—the Problem Today. *J. A. M. A.*, 143:732, June 24, 1950.

(26) Travis, L. E.: *Speech Pathology*. New York, Appleton, 1931.

(27) Gens, G. W.: The Speech Pathologist Looks at the Mentally Deficient Child. *Train. Sch. Bull.*, 48:19, 1951.

(28) Marie, P.: *Semaine Medicale*. 21, 42:48, 1906.

(29) Wechsler, I. S.: *A Textbook of Clinical Neurology*. Philadelphia, W. B. Saunders Co., 1947.

(30) Freeman, G., and Lukens, J.: A Speech and Language Program for Mentally Handicapped Children. *J. Speech & Hearing Disorders*, 27:285, August, 1962.

(31) *Speech for the Retarded Child, A Teacher's Handbook*. New York, Board of Education, 1958-1959 series.

Chapter 11

VOICE DISORDERS

SPEECH AND VOICE

Although speech and voice are associated in many minds as identical, they are separate aspects of the act of speaking. Some people say, "He has a foreign voice," meaning that the speaker has a foreign accent or a foreign form of pronunciation rather than a foreign voice. One hears, "I can tell by his voice that he's a Southerner." What the speaker here means is that, by the sounds uttered, the person reveals characteristics of Southern speech.

Speech is a series of symbolic sound utterances in the form of words, structured into phrases and sentences appropriate to the language being spoken. Voice, on the other hand, is composed of tones caused by vibration of the vocal cords. There may be speech without voice, the whisper, or there may be voice without speech, the inarticulate sounds of the infant. Human speech is, however, made up of a combination of articulate sounds in words, and voice appropriate to the speaker and to the thought expressed.

VOICE IN SPEECH AND SONG

Earlier chapters have described in detail the anatomy and physiology of the speech and vocal mechanisms. Although the physiological actions for speech and song are identical, there are many differences between speaking and singing. In speech, the range of the voice is more limited and the individual notes are not sustained. Pitch, stress, and intonation are used in accordance with the composition of words that the speaker wishes to use in his communication. Furthermore, the difference in the relative importance of vowels and consonants is less marked in speech.

In song, contrasted to speech, the individual notes are sustained and the range of the voice is much greater. Vowels, which carry the musical tone, are of greater relative importance than consonants. Furthermore, in singing, a definite key, pitch, and melody are designated. In other words, in song, the composer indicates exactly how the voice is to be used. In speech, however, the speaker is the composer. Therefore, he uses his voice as his ideas dictate.

NORMAL RESPIRATION AND RESPIRATION FOR SPEECH

Karlin points out differences between normal, quiet respiration and respiration for speech as follows:

Normal Respiration	*Respiration for Speech*
1. Expiration time equals that of inspiration.	1. Expiration time exceeds that of inspiration.
2. Respiration is automatic and involuntary.	2. Respiration is partly under the control of the will.
3. A relatively small amount of air is used.	3. A large amount of air is used.
4. Breathing takes place through the nose.	4. Breathing takes place through the nose and mouth.

EVOLUTION OF THE VOCAL MECHANISM

Negus (1), in his work on the mechanism of the larynx, states that originally this organ was evolved as a valve to guard the entrance to the lungs, and to regulate inspiration and expiration. In the course of further evolution, the larynx, by effecting a firm closure of the glottis, insured a fixed thorax. This provided a firm attachment for the muscles of the arms and shoulder girdle, which was a great advantage for the primates.

For some time the use of the false vocal cords in speech production has been questioned. The false vocal cords are located directly above the true vocal cords. It was thought that their function was to provide protection and an air-tight cover for the vocal cords. Lately it has been shown that during speech, they produce a small cavity, of variable resonance, immediately above the vocal cords. This cavity, together with the fixed cavity of the trachea, assists the action of the vocal cords in securing the required frequency of pulsations in the air column.

NORMAL VOICE

An effective voice is one which attracts no undue attention to itself. It is appropriate to the age and sex of the speaker. In a three-year-old, one cannot always tell by listening to the voice whether a boy or girl is speaking. With increasing age, vocal differences in the sexes become more marked.

An effective speaking voice is pleasant, but the enjoyment of such a voice is passive. The effective voice should neither interfere with, nor distract from, meaning. Rather it should enhance the intended communication.

Objective Characteristics of the Normal Voice

The effective voice should have adequate and *controlled volume*. The speaker should use as much volume as the occasion demands. All members of an audience should hear the voice easily without experiencing a sense of strain or shouting on the part of the speaker. Volume should also vary in accordance with the content of the communication.

A normal voice should also be varied in *pitch*. This should change according to the intellectual and emotional content of the communication. Pitch should also be appropriate to, and in accordance with, the language spoken.

A normal voice should have clear *tone quality*. It should be free from harshness, breathiness, nasality, or strained, hoarse quality.

TYPES OF VOICE DISORDERS

Any departure from normal voice quality is called *dysphonia*. Complete loss of voice is termed *aphonia*. These deficiencies may be due to *organic* or *functional* causes.

Organic Voice Disorders

The organic voice disorders found in children may be directly due to laryngeal involvement or to abnormalities in other areas of speech production. Thus, the anatomical malformations of cleft palate, the neuromuscular abnormalities found in cerebral palsy and bulbar polio, and abnormalities of the resonators, can all contribute toward departures from the normal voice quality of the child.

Laryngeal Abnormalities

The first type of organic voice disorder to be discussed, is due to *congenital* laryngeal abnormalities. One of these is *webbing* between the vocal cords. Webs of the larynx usually unite the cords at their anterior portions. Various explanations have been offered for this condition. One theory states that webs may arise from an intra-uterine infection. Another more likely cause is expounded in the "fusion theory" of incomplete separation of the vocal cords. Early in their development, the primitive vocal cords were adherent to each other. According to the fusion theory, a partial separation of the original functional structure would leave congenital bands or webs.

Laryngitis is probably the most common acute infectious cause of abnormality in voice quality. Chronic syphilitic or tuberculous involvement of the larynx can also produce a lack of flexibility of the vocal cords. This results in a failure of the proper vibratory mechanism so necessary for the production of the normal voice. Although laryngitis is frequently due to an organic etiology, it also may arise from intense vocal abuse such as prolonged shouting.

There are other causes of hoarseness or aphonia in children which are organic and involve the larynx as part of a more generalized neuromuscular or endocrinologic abnormality. Damage to the central nervous system resulting in *cerebral palsy* or *bulbar poliomyelitis* may result in profound changes in voice production. Hoarseness may also result from endocrine changes found in children exhibiting *hypothyroidism* and *hyperpituitarism*.

Vocal Defects Due to Abnormalities in the Resonators

Nasality—(Hyperrhinolalia). Nasality as a functional habit of speech is discussed later in this chapter. Another form of nasality is due to a malformation of the oral cavity known as *cleft palate.* Cleft palate is discussed in detail in a later chapter.

In cases of cleft palate, the hard palate, which separates the buccal from the nasal cavity, is open. The hard palate has not grown together prenatally. If the cleft extends from the upper lip, across the upper gum ridge, across the hard palate, and down the soft palate, then one has cleft lip as well as cleft palate. Thus, there are varying degrees of malformation. Because of an opening in the hard palate, and because of accompanying malformation of the soft palate, the air from the larynx passes from the mouth up into the nose. Breath, coming through the larynx passes out through the mouth and the nose at the same time. The resulting voice is extremely nasal and breathy. This quality is so marked that it calls attention to itself, interferes with communication, and is, therefore, a severe handicap.

Denasality—(Hyporhinolalia). Denasality is defined as having too little nasal resonance. This is caused by obstructions or congestion in the nasal passage. *Adenoids, deviated nasal septum,* or *neoplasms* may make it difficult, even when the nasopharynx is opened by the action of the soft palate, for air to pass out through the nose.

If the obstruction is in the posterior part of the nasal cavity, as in the case of adenoids, the nasal sounds *m, n,* and *ng,* are pronounced *b, d,* and *g* respectively. Thus "spring has come" would sound like "sprig has cub." If, on the other hand, the obstruction is in the anterior nares, there is usually a muffling of the *m, n,* and *ng,* and a tendency for all other sounds to be nasalized.

Allergies, sinusitis, and severe head colds cause the same kind of denasalized voice. In these cases the nasal cavity, which is used in forming the nasal consonants, cannot function normally.

Vocal Defects Due to Other Organic Causes

Voice of the Deaf or Hard of Hearing. The typical vocal pattern of the child with a hearing loss is monotonous. It is lacking in change of pitch, stress, and volume. The intonation pattern, with its rise and fall and glides, is missing. The result is a strange vocal quality that is also lacking in resonance. Since the deaf child cannot imitate the voices of speakers around him, and since he cannot monitor his own speech, he is completely unaware of how the human voice sounds in others and of his own voice quality as well.

If the hearing loss occurs after speech has been acquired, the voice may be too loud or too soft at times, but it will usually have the change in pitch and volume that is heard in the normal voice.

Functional Voice Disorders

Functional voice disorders of youth include *mutational voice disturbance*, dysphonias caused by *poor habits* of vocalization, and dysphonias resulting from *neurotic* tendencies. Also included in this category are changes in the voice due to *singer's nodes*, *vocal polyps*, and *contact ulcers*, although the latter two are quite rare in children.

Mutational Voice Disturbances

The voice, during puberty, at the age of thirteen or fourteen in boys, and eleven or twelve in girls, undergoes remarkable changes. The larynx grows rapidly during this period. In boys at puberty, the lower pitch limit falls an entire octave, and the upper limit falls about one-sixth of an octave. In girls, the lower limit falls about one-third of an octave and the upper limit rises slightly. The sudden growth of the larynx causes difficulty in controlling the voice.

Endocrine glandular anomalies in sexual maturation exercise a marked influence on the changes in the larynx. Thus, an adult male may have a falsetto voice. On the other hand, this type of voice may be psychogenic in origin.

According to Brodnitz (2), "Mutation, the change of voice, is the most important landmark in the vocal history of an individual." He states further that "modern psychiatry has taught us to understand the impact of childhood and adolescence on the emotional problems of the adult . . . In many cases the pattern of adult vocal behavior has become fixed during the pubertal change of the voice."

Nasality

One of the most common forms of functional dysphonia is a quality of voice that is due to expiration of the breath through the nose and mouth at the same time. This manner of speech causes nasality which may vary in quality from slight to very marked. As has been seen in the chapter on articulation, there are only three sounds in English that are pronounced by allowing the air column to pass out through the nose. These sounds consist of *m, n,* and *ng.* In these cases the mouth cavity is closed so that exhaled air is routed out through the nasopharynx and finally, out through the nose. When the lips are placed together and the sound *m* is prolonged as in humming, air passes out through the nose only. The resulting voice is not an unpleasant one, since the wave front is directed through one passage only.

Nasality is due to the audible passage of the air column through the nose at a time other than during the articulation of *m, n,* and *ng.* It is possible for a small amount of air to pass through the nose without being perceived by the ear of the listener.

The soft palate is raised to close off the nasopharnyx. The degree of the closure varies in accordance with the articulation of certain sounds. In sounding the vowel *ah* as in *father,* for example, the soft palate is not so strongly contracted and raised as it is for the vowels *oo* as in *food,* and *ee* as in *see.* The closure of the nasopharynx is also assisted by the contraction of the superior pharyngeal muscle, producing an elevation of the posterior pharyngeal wall known as *Passavant's cushion.* In the closure of the nasopharyngeal port, Passavant's cushion functions in concert with the velum or soft palate.

If the speaker does not close off the passage between the oral and nasal cavities, the resulting voice quality is both piercing and monotonous. Above all, it is extremely fatiguing for the listener. Speaking with the soft palate lowered is frequently a habit. The speaker is unaware of the undesirable quality of his voice. One objective way to convince him of the unpleasantness of his voice, is to have him record his speech on tape and to play it back. As the speaker listens to his own speech, a look of complete astonishment, even disbelief appears on his face. It is obvious that he was totally unaware of his faulty voice.

Children often imitate a nasal voice if it is part of their early speech environment. The normal voice of a child is light, relatively high, and somewhat lacking in resonance. The natural childish voice is free from nasality. If nasality is imitated from the environment by the child, it may remain with him during his entire life. It is important, therefore, for the parents to use good voice quality in the home.

It is interesting to note that in some communities where English is spoken, nasality is a speech characteristic. Since this voice quality is used by the entire community, the children do not hear it in themselves or in others.

Breathiness

This quality is characterized by a lack of clear tone. It is caused by the passage of too much air between the vocal cords. The result is a voice that is part whisper and part tone. A temporary breathiness may be caused by being "out of breath" after having run a long distance or upstairs to deliver a spoken message. The speaker finds that, because he needs to take deep breaths and to release them rapidly as he speaks, his voice is a half whisper because of the excess air escaping as he talks. The chronically breathy voice is often due to shyness or insecurity on the part of the child.

Other Types of Functional Voice Defects

The *monotonous* voice is due to withdrawal from communication, shyness, or physical weakness. Very often monotony is due to indifference or lack of interest. Children may use very varied voices in the playground, but monotonous voices in the schoolroom. Proper motivation in school should improve the voice quality for communication in class.

The *strident* voice is characterized by over-loudness, harshness, and sometimes by hoarseness. The strident voice may also have a nasal quality. This type of voice is due to tension and emotional stress. It, too, can be a habit of which the speaker is unaware. The strident voice, if it is used constantly, often causes nodules on the vocal cords and physical fatigue.

Children, excited at play, use strident voices. If strident voices are heard in the home, a sense of tension and a lack of harmony is produced, which will affect the emotional attitude of the child.

Singer's Nodes, Vocal Polyps, Contact Ulcers

The three entities of *singer's nodes, vocal polyps,* and *contact ulcers* have both functional and organic components that contribute toward voice abnormalities. In all these conditions, the pathogenesis of the disorder is functional, while the resulting abnormality is organic.

Chorditis nodosa, or singer's nodules, is the most common of these causes of dysphonia. The nodes form as a result of misuse of the voice. They are likened to callous growths on the hands or feet due to constant irritation. These growths on the vocal cords are due to excessive tension of the extrinsic and intrinsic muscles of the larynx during the act of singing or speaking. Although juvenile nodes are more common in men, the incidence is reversed in the adult age group.

The presence of these nodes affects the voice in the following two ways. First, some dysphonia results from deflection of the air column by the nodules. Second, dampening of the vibratory mechanism of the vocal cords takes place. During phonation of notes on the lower register, the cords are more widely separated. Comparatively little dysphonia is experienced since the opposing nodes do not touch. Even when the higher register is attempted, the posterior third of each cord is closely approximated and not in use. The voice, therefore, is not greatly affected. When the middle register is attempted, however, the vocal cords vibrate over their entire length. In this case, the nodes touch and interfere with vibration. The result is severe hoarseness or aphonia. Thus, the presence of singer's nodes has a marked affect on the voice, since it involves the most commonly used middle frequency range.

Vocal polyps, or polypoid thickening of the vocal cords, is another organic abnormality due to functional misuse of the voice in a manner similar to that found in patients exhibiting singer's nodules. Brodnitz (3) states that less recurrence of polyps is found in cases treated surgically *combined* with subsequent voice therapy, than in those cases treated by surgery alone. Thus, proper instruction in the use of the voice to avoid extreme tension of the laryngeal musculature, is a necessary prophylactic measure.

Contact ulcers, another form of laryngeal abnormality, may form because of abuse of the voice or as a result of dust and

TABLE IX

Diagnosis	No. Cases	%	Sex M	Sex F	Mean Age
Hyperfunct.	188	24.8	102	86	39.2
Prim. hyperfunct.	33	4.4	20	13	32.4
Juv. nodules	29	3.9	17	12	9.9
Adult nodules	119	15.9	17	102	29.8
Polyps	159	21.4	80	79	43.6
Polyp. thickening	73	9.8	26	47	49.4
Contact ulcers	33	4.4	30	3	48.7
Mutational	42	5.7	38	4	23.4
Hemorrhages (cords)	18	2.5	7	11	29.3
Aphonia	23	3.0	3	20	31.3
Spast. dysphon.	31	4.2	13	18	47.4
Total	748	100.0	353	395	35.8

Table IX. Functional Voice Disorders. From Friedrich Brodnitz's Goals, Results, and Limitations of Vocal Rehabilitation, *Archives of Otolaryngology*, 77:148, 1963. Courtesy of American Medical Association, Chicago, Illinois.

TABLE X

Diagnosis	No. Cases	%	Sex M	Sex F	Mean Age
Paralysis	38	16.7	16	22	39.5
Hypernasality	18	7.8	10	8	14.3
Ventric. voice	9	3.9	6	3	58.2
Leukoplakia	14	6.2	14	—	51.3
Papilloma (adults)	9	3.9	6	3	50.4
Granuloma (post-anesth.)	9	3.9	5	4	48.8
Sulcus vocalis	4	1.7	4	—	32.4
Asymmetry, larynx	7	3.1	6	1	42.3
Webs	7	3.1	5	2	44.6
Laryng. trauma	9	3.9	6	3	28.8
Hormonal	12	5.2	—	12	37.3
Glossectomy	6	2.6	6	—	60.3
Carcinoma, larynx	38	16.6	37	1	59.2
Laryngectomy	49	21.4	42	7	61.3
Total	229	100.0	163	66	44.6

Table X. Organic Voice Disorders. From Friedrich Brodnitz's Goals, Results, and Limitations of Vocal Rehabilitation, *Archives of Otolaryngology*, 77:148, 1963. Courtesy of American Medical Association, Chicago, Illinois.

other irritants to the vocal cords. Symptoms of this difficulty include marked hoarseness or complete loss of voice.

In 1963, Brodnitz (3) tabulated the causes of both functional and organic voice disorders occurring in a large series of cases (Tables IX and X). Although examination of these tables shows that the mean age of all the voice abnormalities occurred in adults, it is significant that conditions classified as functional voice disorders arose in younger age groups than the organic disorders.

TREATMENT OF VOICE DISORDERS

The treatment of voice abnormalities depends upon the cause of the difficulty. It is essential for the patient to have first a laryngoscopic examination by an otolaryngologist. An endocrinologist must be consulted if a glandular disturbance, for example, hypothyroidism, causes hoarseness. It is important to remember, however, that even with medical and surgical diagnosis and treatment, a habit of voice will not always disappear by itself. Thus, a voice specialist should be consulted following medical therapy.

VOICE TREATMENT FOR ORGANIC
ANOMALIES OF THE RESONATORS

Cleft Palate

The surgeon is often successful in closing a cleft in the child born with *cleft palate*. A prosthetic device called an obturator is often used when the surgeon cannot repair the cleft. Two children's ad interim speech-aids are shown in Figure 36. They are useful in covering the hard palate, thus closing the cleft. A bulb, as part of the prosthetic appliance, is also useful to form a closure for the nasopharynx. Further reference to the treatment of cleft palate is made in a later chapter.

Speech therapy is imperative in cases of anomalies in the resonators due to cleft palate. Instruction in both voice and articulation is indicated. Speech work is required following surgical treatment, prosthetic fitting, and/or orthodontia. Better speech will not emerge of itself simply because of physical

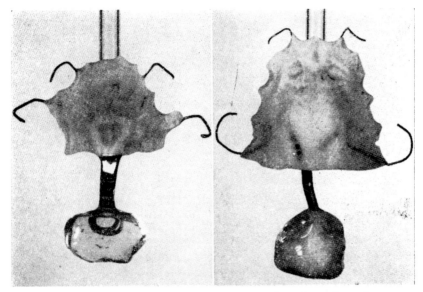

Figure 36. Two children's ad interim speech-aids. These have bent-wire clasps that are retained by lugs soldered on orthodontic bands which have been fitted to the deciduous teeth. Courtesy of the Cleft Palate Center and Training Program of the Professional Colleges and the Division of Services for Crippled Children of the University of Illinois, Chicago, Illinois.

changes in the oral cavity. Surgery, prosthesis, and orthodontia help immeasurably to make it possible for the child to speak more adequately. However, the child does not do so spontaneously, without speech instruction.

Nasal Obstruction or Congestion

If the voice is denasalized because of *adenoids* or *nasal polyps,* it follows that after surgical removal the child has to be taught proper breathing for speech. This consists of instruction in both nose and mouth breathing instead of the previous mouth breathing only.

It is necessary for parents to consult an allergist if *allergies* and *sinusitis* cause a denasalized, hoarse, and breathy voice in the child. In addition, voice instruction often helps to improve the vocal quality of the voice, even though the allergic condition is present or may become chronic. A head cold may also cause the same variations in voice as sinusitis. When the child no longer has the cold, a normal voice should return.

HEARING LOSS

The speech and voice teacher is essential in cases of vocal defects due to *deafness* or hearing loss. This is especially true for children with mutism, a condition due to loss of hearing before speech is learned. When hearing is impaired after speech has been acquired, the voice and speech are usually adequate.

SPEECH THERAPY FOR FUNCTIONAL VOICE DISORDERS

Weiss (4), Froeschels, and Brodnitz (2) have made large contributions in the field of *mutational voice disorders*. They have brought the pitch of the male voice down to normal levels in cases where voice mutation has been faulty or incomplete. Brodnitz (2) states that the pressure test provides "new proof of the psychological character of postmutational voice disturbances." Brodnitz summarizes by saying that "pressure on the thyroid cartilage during phonation produces, in normal voices, an initial lowering of the voice. In patients with postmutational voice disturbances of the mutational falsetto and of the incomplete mutation type, a paradoxic pattern of initial pitch rise on pressure was observed. The observation is interpreted as a confirmation of the psychogenic character of these voice disturbances."

Many functional voice defects are due to personality traits or to neurotic tendencies. Training in the proper use of the soft palate to close off the nasal port, ear training, and relaxation are essential elements in cases of *functional nasality*.

The *breathy voice,* if there is no organic cause, needs building of tone through exercises and practice. Children having this problem often gain confidence through practice. Ear training is essential in all cases.

The speaker with a *monotonous voice* is in need of group speech practice. Choral speaking and singing are often beneficial. Exercises in appropriate intonation and stress for variety in pitch and volume make the speaker aware of the logical value of change of voice during communication.

The *strident* speaker needs instruction in relaxation and release of tension. Speech and voice instruction that stress the relaxed approach to communication help this kind of speaker. Since this type of voice is due to personality traits, it is essential to use a psychological approach to treatment.

In the case of functional voice disorders, the phoniatrist has to surmount the child's unconscious resistance toward therapy. This is true inasmuch as the speaker with a functional voice defect does not welcome any deep-rooted change in his personality traits. Failure to practice exercises, and resistance to suggestions are often causes for lack of improvement in the child with functional voice disorders.

If the cause of the voice defect is a functional abnormality in the larynx itself, a laryngologist must be seen. If surgery is necessary for removal of laryngeal nodules or polyps, post-operative treatment by a phoniatrist is imperative. Since singer's nodes are caused by misuse of the voice, they are likely to return unless the speaker is trained to use his voice properly. The person who suffers from hoarseness due to singer's nodes should refrain from singing and loud speech, should learn proper means of voice support, and above all, should learn how to avoid tension of the muscles governing the voice mechanism. In the case of contact ulcers, complete vocal rest for six months or a year is recommended.

TREATMENT FOR THE LARYNGECTOMIZED

Complete laryngectomy is extremely rare in children, although isolated reports do appear in the literature. Its inclusion in a book concerned with speech disorders in children is justified, however, since voice rehabilitation is of such paramount concern following surgical removal of the larynx.

Complete laryngectomy is the treatment of choice for patients having cancer of the larynx. It is also performed in certain selected cases of severe neck trauma, such as was sustained during World War II. It is extremely necessary, therefore, to provide a means of restoring the voice to these people. Many of the instructors are laryngectomees themselves.

Normal speech depends upon three factors. These include: respiration, governed by the lungs and diaphragm; phonation,

dependent upon a normal, intact larynx; and articulation, performed by structures in the oropharyngeal cavity. After laryngectomy, the expired air, so necessary for the production of
speech, is prevented from passing out from the lungs into the
mouth because of the closure of the normal passageway. Thus,
air travels to and from the lungs by means of the artificial opening provided by the neck surgery. This method of air intake, although providing for adequate respiration so necessary for life,
cannot be used for the production of speech. Furthermore, there
can be little vibration of sounds by the outgoing air column,
since the vocal cords have been removed.

In buccal speech, only the voiceless consonants are actually
After laryngectomy, patients often develop speech which makes
use of the principle of whispering. In the absence of the normal
air passage and the vocal cords, they use the air in the mouth to
form voiceless sounds. This type of communication is called *buccal speech.*

In buccal speech, only the voiceless consonants are actually
articulated, *p, f, th* (as in *thin*), *t, s, sh, ch,* and *k.* Other sounds
are formed by the lips and tongue and are "read" by the listener.
Buccal speech can be understood by the family, but is not useful
for business or social intercourse. Naturally, it cannot carry over
a telephone.

The Artificial Larynx

The *artificial larynx* was an early device to provide the necessary vibrations that are lost due to the removal of the vocal cords.
It is infrequently used today. One end of a tube is placed over
the surgically created opening in the trachea. The other end is
placed in the mouth. Within the tube is a reed which vibrates
when air from the lungs passes over it. There are two outlets for
air in the artificial larynx. One provides for normal respiration.
The other is used for speaking. When the respiratory outlet is
open, air will by-pass the vibrator and no sound will be heard.
For speech, the finger is placed over this orifice, causing the air
to pass over the second outlet containing the vibrator. The vibrating air then passes through the tube to the other opening located
in the mouth. Here, the air is formed into articulate sounds. A

patient can learn to produce speech with very little practice when using this device.

There are many disadvantages to this method of producing speech. First, the device has to be inserted and removed. Second, it is cosmetically undesirable. Third, the artificial larynx can be easily damaged. Fourth, one hand is always occupied while speaking. Last, the device has to be cleaned very carefully. Furthermore, a metallic quality to the voice is produced which has little variation in pitch.

An electrically operated voice box has been developed which consists of an electrically driven vibrator. This mechanism is placed against the throat. Vibrations are transmitted through the walls of the throat and up into the mouth where they are articulated into sounds for speech. Thus, the cumbersome use of a tube in the mouth to provide vibrations is not necessary.

Esophageal Speech

Following laryngectomy, one should first attempt to teach esophageal speech before resorting to any of the previously mentioned devices. Although the artificial larynx is an improvement over buccal speech, it does not form the most desirable means of language communication following removal of the larynx. At present, *esophageal speech* is the best form of speech rehabilitation for the laryngectomee.

Esophageal speech is more natural in quality than buccal or prosthetic laryngeal speech since it does not require the use of an appliance. Training develops the ability to swallow air, hold it in the esophagus and expel it in the form of a controlled "belch." Brodnitz (5) states that "the vibration of air that is necessary for phonation is produced by squeezing the interrupting air through a pseudoglottis, i.e., closely approximated mucous membranes which act as vicarious vocal cords." West (6) suggests that many people who are said to be using esophageal speech are actually employing *pharyngeal speech*. In this case, "the pseudolarynx is the pair of cricopharyngeal muscles."

McDonald (7) states that the belches used for esophageal speech may be formed into "intelligible and esthetically satisfactory speech" by the resonating and articulating structures. Mc-

Donald believes that a successfully rehabilitated patient should be able to "swallow air inconspicuously and in sufficient quantity to produce phrases consisting of several words. He should be able to vary the pitch and intensity of his voice to some extent and should be able to talk for long periods without tiring."

Brodnitz (3) reports that of forty-nine patients referred for training in esophageal speech, twenty-four learned to speak with satisfactory sound and speed; thirteen developed esophageal voice, but were still handicapped by lack of fluency. Of the remaining twelve cases, eight gave up the training after brief attempts. Four were fitted with an artificial aid. Brodnitz states that these results parallel those reported in the literature.

Esophageal-pharyngeal speech can be taught by making use of an ordinary whistle. Gardner (8) states that the patient can learn to impound air in the mouth in order to blow a whistle. Another technique makes use of the *stop* or *plosive* sounds to impound air. A plosive consonant is formed by stopping the air completely and releasing it suddenly. The consonant *t*, for example, is formed by placing the tip of the tongue on the upper gum ridge and lowering it suddenly. The tip of the tongue holds the air in the mouth until the tongue is suddenly lowered. Thus, the laryngectomee learns to keep a supply of air in the mouth for later use in forming sounds.

After he has learned to trap air to blow a whistle using the plosive sound *t*, the whistle is removed and the patient practices making the *t* movement with the lips closed. Next, the back of the tongue is lifted and the throat is relaxed causing the air to be injected into the pharynx where, according to West, the cricopharyngeal muscles may act as a pseudolarynx. Thus, the esophagus or the pharynx may act as a pseudolarynx.

Following practice with the plosive *t*, the patient learns to use the other plosives *d, p, b, k,* and *g* for providing a supply of air in the pharynx. These plosives also leave a residuum of unused air that can be conserved for succeeding sounds. Thus, the patient builds up a system for storing and using impounded air in the mouth for speech.

EVALUATION OF TREATMENT OF VOICE DISORDERS

One may state that there are many steps in voice rehabilitation of the child. Medical examination, speech and voice exercises (unless vocal rest is indicated), recordings of the voice, ear training and practice exercises must be performed frequently in order to obtain good results.

Brodnitz (3) states that "the difficulty in the evaluation of the results of voice therapy is that no simple yardsticks exist to determine the success of the treatment . . . The trained ear of the phoniatrist is still the best means of determining the results of vocal rehabilitation."

REFERENCES

(1) Negus, V. E.: *The Mechanism of the Larynx.* London, Wm. Heinemann, Ltd., 1929.

(2) Brodnitz, F. S.: The Pressure Test in Mutational Voice Disturbances. *Ann. Otol. Rhin. & Laryng.* 67:235, March, 1958.

(3) Brodnitz, F. S.: Goals, Results, and Limitations of Vocal Rehabilitation. *Arch. Otolaryng.,* 77:148, February, 1963.

(4) Weiss, D. A.: The Pubertal Change of the Human Voice (Mutation). *Fol. Phoniatr.,* 2:126, 1950.

(5) Brodnitz, F. S.: *Vocal Rehabilitation.* 2nd Edition. Home Study Course Manual. American Academy of Ophthalmology and Otolaryngology, Rochester, Minnesota, 1961.

(6) West, R.: Personal Communication to the Authors.

(7) McDonald, E. T.: *The Rehabilitation of the Laryngectomized.* Chicago, National Society for Crippled Children & Adults, 1949.

(8) Gardner, W. H.: The Whistle Technique in Esophageal Speech. *J. Speech & Hearing Dis.,* 27:187, May, 1962.

Chapter 12

HEARING PROBLEMS

O<small>NE OF</small> the causes for delay in the development of speech in childhood is either a partial hearing loss or total deafness. It is advisable to define the terms used in the discussion of sound before describing the various types of hearing loss.

THE PROPERTIES OF SOUND

Sound waves carry vibrations of various frequencies. *Frequency* is defined as the number of vibrations or cycles occurring in a unit of time. The frequency determines the nature of the sound perceived by the listener. The range of frequencies most important in understanding speech is from 300 to 3,000 cycles per second (cps). A hearing loss within a certain frequency range causes lack of sensitivity to certain sounds.

Threshold of hearing refers to the least amount of sound necessary to arouse auditory sensation in a normal ear. Best and Taylor (1) state that sounds may differ from one another in three ways. These include *intensity, pitch,* and *quality (timbre)*.

Sound intensity and *loudness* are not synonymous terms. Sound intensity refers to the energy of the sound waves. It is a purely physical value and may be independent of the auditory sensation. Loudness refers to the auditory sensation received by the listener. Loudness of sound depends upon the number of fibers in the acoustic nerve that have been stimulated. West (2) states that this may be a function of the stapedius and tensor tympani muscles. When there are two sounds having the same intensity but different frequency, one may be louder than the other. Since the intensity refers to the energy of the sound wave, it is proportional to the amplitude of these waves.

Pitch is that property of sound which enables the listener to place a tone at a definite level in the musical scale. It depends mainly on the vibration frequency, that is, upon the number of cycles per second falling upon the ear.

Quality or *timbre* is that property of sound by which one distinguishes between two tones of the same pitch and intensity, e.g., the note of a violin from a bugle note. Quality is determined by the wave form. Sounds can be classified into *noises* and *musical tones.*

DEFINITION OF HEARING

Hearing is that function of the ear and brain which translates sound impulses into perceptible tones. The central nervous system is capable of gathering, combining, and transforming sound impulses received from the external acoustic meatus into comprehensible language. The anatomy of the hearing mechanism has already been discussed in an earlier chapter.

The exact site of frequency analysis of sound is still a matter of dispute. Many authorities believe that the cochlea is concerned with sound discrimination. Others feel that frequency analysis of sound is the function of the brain. The *Helmholtz Resonance Theory* states that the cochlea possesses a series of resonators, each tuned to a different frequency. This theory postulates that the shorter fibers of the basilar membrane near the oval window respond to higher frequencies, while the larger fibers near the apex are sensitive to lower frequencies. The *Rutherford Telephone Theory* states that the brain governs the function of sound analysis. According to Rutherford, the role of the cochlea is that of a telephone transmitter, transforming sounds into nerve impulses of the same frequency. The analysis of these nerve impulses takes place, according to this theory, in the cerebral cortex. Rutherford considers the basilar membrane to be simply a converter which transforms mechanical sound into nerve impulses.

HEARING LOSS AND DEAFNESS

The *hard of hearing* child refers to one who, although he has impaired hearing, is still able to develop speech and communicate with others through auditory means. *The deafened* child is one who has lost a significant portion of his hearing after having developed normal speech and language. The *deaf* child is one whose hearing loss is of such severity that even with powerful amplification, he will still depend primarily on non-auditory means for communication.

All three of the previously mentioned terms refer to broad categories. The question is still undecided as to the exact place where the line should be drawn between loss of hearing and deafness.

ORGANIC CAUSES OF HEARING LOSS

The organic etiology of deafness can be broken down into three categories, depending upon the anatomical site of the defect. These include: *conductive* or *transmission* hearing loss, *sensorineural* or *perceptive* loss, and *mixed* impairment.

Conductive Hearing Impairment

A conductive or transmission hearing loss may be defined as impaired hearing resulting from faulty sound transmission through the external or middle ear. This may be due to obstructive phenomena in the external ear or to disease or defects in the middle ear.

Congenital abnormalities of a developmental nature may involve the external ear. *Traumatic* perforation of the tympanic membrane as a result of children playing with foreign bodies such as pencils, forms another broad group. *Cerumen* and other foreign substances in the external acoustic meatus of children may be responsible for hearing loss. *Obstruction* of the *Eustachian tube* caused by enlarged *tonsils* and *adenoids* may impair sound conduction through the middle ear. In this case, there is failure of the Eustachian tube to maintain communication between the nasopharynx and the middle ear.

A *serous otitis media* is a common childhood infection that produces at least a temporary impairment of sound conduction through the middle ear. In this case, an upper respiratory infection causes engorgement of the nasal mucosa and obstruction and congestion in the Eustachian tubes. Decreased aeration of the middle ear follows, resulting in transudation of serous fluid into the middle ear cavity. While an acute otitis media usually causes only temporary impairment of hearing, the subacute and chronic forms are responsible for progressive hearing loss due to fibrous adhesions which limit the movement of the ossicular chain of the middle ear.

Otosclerosis is a common cause of a conductive hearing loss which is progressive in nature. There is an hereditary as well as a familial component to this disease. Although otosclerosis does not occur during childhood, it is said to have its inception in late adolescence. Its pathogenesis can be found in osseous changes commencing in the outer wall of the labyrinth, particularly in the neighborhood of the oval window. Limitation of movement of the stapes results. Thus, one finds impaired bone conduction via the ossicular chain of the middle ear. In addition, there is degeneration of the hair cells of the organ of Corti in the advanced stages, producing sensorineural as well as conductive involvement.

In otosclerosis, the progressive loss of hearing is especially pronounced for low tones. In fact, in cases of chronic ear disease, including otitis media, the child usually experiences a greater loss of hearing in the lower and middle frequency range. In sensorineural deafness, the impairment is mainly for the higher tones.

Paracusis Willisii is characterized by the ability of the hard-of-hearing person to hear better in the presence of loud surrounding noise. It occurs in cases of conductive loss of fairly high degree. Whether it is a real phenomenon is a controversial question. Some investigators believe that the speaker unconsciously raises his voice to drown out the surrounding noise. Thus, the person who is deafened is benefited by the increased loudness of the conversation. Another possible explanation may be that strong vibrations of the surrounding noise set the previously fixed ossicular chain of the middle ear in motion, thus enabling these bones to regain their responsiveness to more complex sounds.

Sensorineural Hearing Impairment

Sensorineural or perceptive hearing impairment results from an abnormality in the organ of Corti or in the acoustic nerve. It may also arise from disease of the labyrinth. The term *central deafness* refers to impaired acoustic perceptibility resulting from lesions in higher centers in the brain. Congenital verbal-auditory agnosia (word deafnesss) is such an example and is discussed in the earlier chapter on aphasia.

A developmental defect of the inner ear may cause deafness. In congenitally deaf children, the semicircular canals may be underdeveloped as well as the cochlear part of the labyrinth. *German measles* is a viral disease that can occur in the mother during the first trimester of pregnancy. It can produce damage to the sensorineural apparatus of the fetus. Damage is produced in the cochlea and auditory pathway central to it. *Inflammatory* bacterial conditions of the labyrinth may cause inadequate hearing.

Extension of localized disease from the middle ear or more generalized infections of the nervous system such as *meningitis* are other examples of conditions producing a perceptive hearing defect. Central nervous system complications from such childhood diseases as *measles, mumps,* and *scarlet fever* are further examples of diseases which can produce sensorineural hearing impairment. Childhood trauma resulting in *fracture* of the base of the skull may also involve the auditory nerve.

It is interesting to note that any childhood disease producing *hyperpyrexia* is capable of producing irreversible damage to the cochlea. Furthermore, *ototoxic. medications* such as streptomycin, dihydrostreptomycin, and neomycin can produce damage to the organ of Corti.

Presbycusis

Presbycusis is defined as changes occurring in the auditory mechanism in the older age groups. Although the subject matter of this book is concerned with children, it is appropriate here to mention advancing age as a cause of hearing impairment. This type of loss occurs often in the high frequency range.

The major pathology in presbycusic hearing loss affects the cochlea and structures central to it. Another very important factor, however, is the slower cerebration of the older person. A time-lag in interpreting sounds that are heard will cause the person of more advanced years to fall behind when listening to a rapidly moving conversation. This alteration in the reaction time is in keeping with the psychological pattern of advancing age.

FUNCTIONAL HEARING IMPAIRMENT

There are three types of functional bases for a hearing loss in a child. First, one may have a psychological accompaniment to a case of an organic hearing defect. Second, there may be a primary functional cause without organic involvement. A third form of non-organic auditory impairment is found in the malingerer.

An increased awareness of the possibility of psychogenic deafness has developed in recent years. In this type of hearing impairment, maladjustment in personality is evidenced in a hearing loss. Much of the literature on this subject indicates that in psychogenic hearing impairment, there is usually some organic loss of hearing. The problem is to measure the extent of the non-organic factor that accompanies the hearing defect.

An important clinical clue to the presence of a non-organic hearing loss is the ability of the child to hear speech at a softer level than is suggested by the pure tone audiogram. An unusually large or an unaccountably small gain in sensitivity with a hearing aid may also be an indication that a psychogenic component exists. A functional hearing loss may also be suspected when there are marked inconsistencies in the child's responses to routine audiometric retesting. Hypnotic suggestion and narcosynthesis are done infrequently in children, but may be attempted to determine the extent of the psychogenic component of a hearing loss. In narcosynthesis, hearing tests are administered while the patient is under the influence of a drug.

The problem of functional hearing disorders has been noted especially in Army and Navy rehabilitation centers. Reports from these sources suggest that of those personnel on active duty referred for hearing problems, ten to twenty per cent were found to have a functional component.

Although Army and Navy investigations of psychogenic hearing impairment are concerned primarily with adults, children may also have emotional bases for lack of acuity in hearing or in the comprehension of speech. It is, therefore, necessary to take these important factors into consideration when investigating the nature and extent of a hearing loss in a child. A further discussion of functional hearing loss in the child is considered in a later chapter on speech disorders in emotional disturbances.

EFFECT OF LOW AND HIGH FREQUENCY LOSS ON SPEECH

The vowel and diphthong sounds have most of their acoustic energy below 1000 cycles. These sounds contribute greatly to the energy and resonance characteristics of speech. Understanding of speech is also determined by the ability to hear consonant sounds. Such sounds have their primary acoustic energy in the high frequencies above 1000 cps. As a group, the consonant sounds are from twelve to twenty decibels softer than the vowels.

Children with low frequency losses due to conductive hearing impairment of sound, have relatively little difficulty in understanding speech, providing its intensity is adequate for them. Their articulation is relatively unaffected by their hearing loss, although they may show some general voice changes. The child with a high frequency loss will have considerable difficulty in the perception and production of high frequency consonants: *s, sh, th, f,* etc. He will have considerable difficulty in differentiating words which are similar except for the consonantal elements, e.g., *sin, tin, pin,* and *fin.*

SYMPTOMS AND SIGNS OF HEARING LOSS

There are certain clues that may indicate auditory impairment in a child. An adequate history and a careful study of a child's behavioral patterns often serve to alert the investigator that a hearing loss may be present. Facial expression, focus of the eyes, and gestures such as nodding or shaking the head, all serve to indicate the reception and comprehension of speech and language through the auditory route. An absence of these factors gained through observation of the child in his normal, everyday environment may provide a reasonable index of suspicion that a hearing loss is present. Furthermore, hearing defects frequently result in changes in behavior. Thus, the child may listen with the head tilted toward one side or he may be restless and inattentive.

The history and physical findings of the otolaryngologist frequently lead to a diagnosis of hearing loss. A history of chronic earache, tinnitus, and aural discharge is of particular significance. Observation of a perforated or injected tympanic membrane is an important finding.

One may suspect a case of impaired hearing if one learns to recognize some of the speech sequelae arising from chronic ear disease. These include: failure to respond to speech in the environment, delayed speech, defects in speech, strange voice quality, and lack of control of volume of the voice. Indeed, when a preschool child exhibits delayed speech, the possibility of a hearing loss must always be seriously entertained.

In children with conductive hearing deficiencies the voice is often subdued in volume. In youngsters with sensorineural impairment the voice may be increased in volume sometimes to an actual shout. It may be noted here that conductive deafness is less serious in its effect upon speech because the child can hear himself speak.

Children who have an undetected hearing loss and who do not understand what is said, are often suspected of being "slow" mentally. The child who is really "slow" but who has no hearing loss, suffers loss of comprehension as a result of poor cerebration or mental deficiency. He will have a low intelligence quotient. Naturally, a child who has both a hearing impairment coupled with mental deficiency, will present a complicated educational problem.

SUBJECTIVE TESTS FOR HEARING

Following a thorough history and physical examination, including evaluation of the child's mental ability, one should perform tests to determine whether or not a hearing loss is present. The watch-tick test and the conversational voice test are among the most simple, although subject to considerable error. They are screening tests of hearing, telling the examiner whether a hearing loss is present or absent. Tuning fork tests and audiometric testing (with pure tones and speech) represent more refined methods of evaluating the kind and degree of hearing loss. Audiometric studies, when properly performed, help to determine the part of the auditory apparatus affected.

Watch-tick and Conversational Voice Tests

For the *watch-tick test,* any watch may be used that can be heard by the average ear at a distance of three feet. The child stands sideways in relation to the examiner with cotton in the untested ear to mask the one not being tested. The watch is placed close to the ear and gradually withdrawn until the child fails to hear the tick. The test is then reversed. Beginning at a distance of thirty-six inches, the examiner brings the watch toward the subject and stops as soon as the child hears the tick. An average of the two tests is made. If the child is unable to hear the ticking at twenty inches, hearing acuity is 20/36.

In the *conversational voice test,* the examiner draws a chalk line twenty feet long on the floor. The child stands at the farther end of this line. The child's back is turned as the examiner says words, numbers, or syllables with ordinary volume to his voice. The youngster should be able to repeat these accurately.

Recent investigations have demonstrated conclusively the serious limitations of these types of auditory screening procedures.

Tuning Fork Tests

Any condition preventing conduction of sound to the inner ear or interfering with the conveyance of nerve impulses to the brain can cause impaired hearing. *Conductive (transmission)* hearing loss refers to an abnormality involving the passage of sound through the external and middle ear. Disease confined to the middle ear affects the transmission of air-conducted sounds only. Conduction through the bones of the skull remains unaltered. *Sensorineural (perceptive)* hearing loss refers to damage to the cochlea, the auditory nerve, or higher areas. In hearing impairment resulting from disease of the inner ear or of the auditory pathway, bone conduction is affected.

Bone conduction measurements play an important role in the differential diagnosis between conductive and perceptive hearing loss. A defect in hearing resulting from bone conduction can be determined by using a vibrating *tuning fork.* The following tuning fork tests are among those employed to differentiate conductive from perceptive deafness.

Rinne's Test

In the *Rinne test,* the vibrating fork is first placed on the mastoid process. When the child states that he no longer can hear its tone by bone conduction, the vibrating tuning fork is then held close to the external acoustic meatus. The normal ear should then continue to hear the fork by air conduction. This is a positive Rinne test and will also be found in persons with perceptive impairments. The test is considered negative if the tuning fork is heard longer by bone conduction. A negative Rinne test is found in persons with conductive impairments.

Weber's Test

The *Weber test* is a useful tuning fork test to determine the type of hearing loss present. It consists of placing the vibrating fork in the midline on the child's head and asking him to state in which ear he hears the tone louder. If there is no auditory impairment, the youngster will hear equally well with both ears. If one ear has a perceptive lesion, the sound will be heard in the *better* ear. If one ear has a conductive defect, the sound will be heard in the *poorer* ear.

Schwabach's Test

Schwabach's test measures the degree of bone conduction loss. The child's bone conduction time is compared with that of the normal examiner. The length of time during which the examiner hears the sound after it becomes inaudible to the patient gives a measure of the bone conduction hearing loss. A child with middle ear deafness hears the sound by bone conduction longer than the examiner, in whose ear the tone is masked by room noises. In perceptive hearing loss, the tone is heard through bone for a shorter time than the normal.

PURE TONE AUDIOMETRY

Audiometric testing is the best and most widely used method for determining severity and kind of hearing loss. The *Pure Tone Audiometer* is an instrument that produces tones of various frequencies. Its frequency range usually extends from 125 to 8,000 cycles per second (cps), whereas its intensity range covers approximately 100 decibels (db). Each tone may be regulated in volume through the use of controls similar to the volume controls

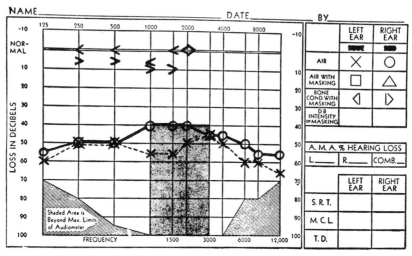

Figure 37. Audiogram showing loss of hearing caused by impairment of the conductive mechanism. Courtesy of The Maico Company, Inc., Minneapolis, Minnesota.

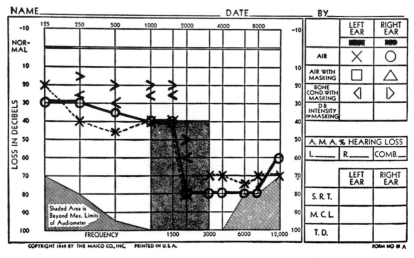

Figure 38. Audiogram showing loss of hearing caused by impairment of the sensorineural mechanism. Courtesy of The Maico Company, Inc., Minneapolis, Minnesota.

on a television or radio set. The intensity of the tone is measured in decibels. A subject who is just able to detect all the frequencies within fifteen decibels has normal threshold and is said to have normal hearing. If the child's threshold of hearing is thirty-five decibels, however, that means that he cannot hear a specific tone unless the intensity or volume of the tone is thirty-five decibels greater than that which is heard by the normal listener. A graph showing the audiometric threshold plotted as a function of frequency is called an *audiogram*. The shape of the audiogram provides valuable information concerning the nature of the hearing loss. Figures 37 and 38 show typical audiograms representing cases of conductive and sensorineural auditory impairment, respectively.

The test for air conduction measures the integrity of the entire auditory system. In the test for bone conduction, vibrations pass through the temporal bone to the inner ear and thus to the organ of Corti where the nerve endings are situated. Thus, the external and middle ear are by-passed. Earphones are used during the air conduction test. A vibrator is placed over the mastoid process in testing bone conduction. The air conduction test provides the examiner with an over-all measure of the child's sensitivity for pure tones. Testing for bone conduction will determine the function of the inner ear and permits the differentiation between conductive and sensorineural impairments.

Both intensity (loudness) and frequency (pitch) are used for evaluating hearing in the aforementioned tests. Normal hearing for a child should be between 250 to 8,000 cps within normal limits. The high frequency sounds in speech are *s, z, sh, zh, th, p, b, t, d, f, v,* and *h.* These speech sounds will not be heard normally by the child who does not hear frequencies over 1,000 cps. For this child, there is an awareness of speech, but he has difficulty in understanding what he hears. Vowels and diphthongs are most audible in this type of hearing loss.

SPEECH AUDIOMETRY

The previously mentioned tests are used to indicate the degree and type of hearing loss for pure tones. Although pure tone audiometry is used to determine the kind of hearing loss sustained, it cannot measure the child's ability to hear and understand speech. It is, therefore, necessary to test the child using appropriate speech stimuli.

The frequencies of greatest importance for the understanding of speech are those located in the middle of the audiometric range. If the hearing of 500, 1000, and 2000 cps is significantly impaired, hearing for speech is also affected. The average hearing loss for these three frequencies usually provides a reasonably close estimate of the hearing loss for speech when the audiometric configuration is essentially flat.

Sensitivity is the ability to detect soft speech. A test for sensitivity tells one how intense speech must be made before the child responds to it. *Discrimination* is the ability to understand audible speech by differentiating among phonetic elements. A test for discrimination tells how well the child recognizes words in speech. In general, a reduction in sensitivity, a so-called "hearing loss," is noted in conductive deafness, whereas difficulty in discrimination is more frequently associated with sensorineural involvement.

Spondaic Words

The speech reception threshold is usually determined by using a list of *spondaic,* or *disyllabic words,* having equal stress on each syllable. The words *baseball* and *railroad* are examples of disyllabic words.

In testing sensitivity with spondaic words, the procedure is to present groups of these words at successively lower intensity levels. The lowest level at which the child can repeat correctly fifty per cent of the words is called "the threshold for speech." The difference between this value and the average threshold for normal listeners represents the child's hearing loss for speech.

Phonetically Balanced Word Lists

Speech discrimination evaluates the child's ability to understand everyday English. The speech one hears varies greatly in intelligibility partly because some phonetic elements are harder to identify than others. Lists of "phonetically balanced" monosyllables have been prepared which reflect the proportion in which they occur in English. Thus, the *Phonetically Balanced Word List* was developed.

In testing with monosyllables, each list is presented to the child at a constant intensity. This procedure is in contrast to testing for sensitivity with spondaic words in which the intensity of the stimulus is varied. The child's "articulation score" on the Phonetically Balanced Word List Test is the per cent of words repeated correctly at the given intensity level. The child's average articulation score for faint (55 db. Sound Pressure Level), normal (70 db. Sound Pressure Level), and loud (85 db. Sound Pressure Level) conversational speech is a useful measure of his ability to hear speech in everyday situations and is referred to as the *Social Adequacy Index*.

OBJECTIVE TESTS FOR HEARING

In cases where patients are unable or unwilling to cooperate in either pure tone or speech audiometry, *the electrodermal reflex* (EDR) and the *electroencephalogram* (EEG) are used. Contrasted to the tests just previously discussed, these two methods for testing hearing do not depend upon the subjective responses of the child. They, therefore, can be used in very young children or in a child who does not have the mental capacity to respond to routine hearing test instructions. EDR and EEG audiometry can be of invaluable assistance for the emotionally disturbed child such as the autistic or schizophrenic youngster who may not subjectively react to auditory stimuli.

Electrodermal Reflex

In the electrodermal (psychogalvanic skin resistance) test, the child is conditioned to expect a mild electric shock whenever he hears a tone. The shock brings forth a sudden, transient change in the electrical resistance of the skin. The tone, representing the conditioned stimulus, comes to have the same effect. The difference in the electrical resistance of the skin represents the electrodermal reflex response. By recording the skin response and noting whether a change occurs when tones are sounded at various levels, one can determine the child's threshold of hearing.

Electroencephalographic Test

In the electroencephalographic test (EEG), there is a change in the electroencephalographic pattern in response to sound. This change in wave pattern occurs in light sleep and is used as an indication that a given tone has been heard. Tones of varying intensities are introduced similar to the procedure for electrodermal reflex audiometry.

Both EDR and EEG audiometry require considerable skill in the interpretation of the records. Although these techniques differentiate between the presence and absence of hearing, they do not make possible the accurate measurement of the hearing loss in all cases. However, since subjective tests for hearing depend upon the variables of interest, attention span, and the reaction time of the child, the more objective tests of EDR and EEG audiometry are important because they reduce the number of unknown variables.

DIAGNOSIS

Hearing in the normal infant is relatively acute a few days after birth. Musical notes may be pleasing to the infant by the age of four months, or even earlier. Many babies are obviously soothed by a soft voice or a lullaby.

A complete medical examination is recommended if a hearing loss is suspected in an infant or a young child. If a child can cooperate in an audiometric examination, an audiogram will indicate the nature and extent of the hearing loss. If a child cannot cooperate in standard audiometric testing, then EDR and EEG audiometry may be attempted.

A hearing disability may cause delay in speech and language development in addition to defects in voice and articulation. An audiogram that shows a loss of more than twenty-five decibels for the speech frequencies in the better ear indicates a definite handicap. Children exhibiting a mild loss will understand speech at close range, but may do poorly at school if they are seated in the rear of the room. Children who show a loss of more than forty decibels are classified as hard of hearing.

A child exhibiting conductive deafness will speak in a soft

voice because his speech sounds louder to him than it does to the listener. A child with sensorineural deafness will often shout in order to hear his own voice.

TREATMENT OF HEARING LOSS

It is important to remember that children with a conductive hearing impairment can often be successfully treated. The loss is frequently reversible. The removal of cerumen as well as the relatively simple procedures of tonsillectomy and adenoidectomy result in regaining previously lost auditory function. The older procedure of fenestration as well as the more recent operation of stapedectomy, have contributed much toward the reversibility of hearing loss in cases of otosclerosis.

When one encounters a sensorineural hearing defect in a child, it is for the most part a very difficult problem to treat. Here, surgery offers little promise for the restitution of hearing. Many times, it is a question of obtaining amplification of sound through the use of a hearing aid as well as making greater use of visual cues in communication.

Suggestions for Speech Therapy

Lack of normal auditory function produces serious delay in the intellectual activity of the child. Luriya and Yudovich (3) state that the child of seven to eight years of age "begins to solve complex problems with the aid of systems of internal verbal connections which have arisen earlier." How can the child who is not equipped with these "systems of internal verbal connections" make up for his loss? How can he be helped to compensate? How can he learn language which has been limited or denied to him because of a significant reduction in hearing sensitivity?

Fortunately, authorities concerned with speech rehabilitation in children, such as pediatricians, otolaryngologists, audiologists, speech clinicians, educators, psychologists, and many other personnel are working to help solve some of these problems. The following discussion contains therapeutic suggestions for the child with a hearing loss.

Use of a Hearing Aid

The audiologist should make his recommendations concerning the use of a hearing aid prior to any formal speech training. The child should be fitted with one, if findings indicate the need. If the child is to have a hearing aid, both he and the parents should receive proper training in the use and care of the device. The audiologist must determine whether greater benefit can be derived from the use of a monaural aid, or a binaural device. In any case, recent advances in audiology, electronics, and acoustic engineering have made hearing aids more and more useful to the hard of hearing and deaf child.

Since the ability to learn language in early childhood is based upon hearing speech in the environment, any device that can sharpen sensitivity will be most helpful in language development.

Planning Speech Therapy

A child should have instruction in speech as early as possible after it is apparent that he has either no speech or is severely handicapped by unintelligible speech. He may receive such instruction at a public or private school for the deaf, or in a university or hospital speech clinic. Teaching should include speech reading, i.e., "reading" speech by watching the speaker.

The speech clinician should prepare an articulation and voice profile for each child. This is accomplished by using standard articulation tests. The profiles will be most helpful in planning an instructional program and in grouping children for work in speech.

The goal of teaching spoken language to the hypacusic child is to increase the intelligibility of oral communication. It is important to remember that intelligibility in speech depends upon elements other than the articulation of sounds alone. Lengthening of sounds where it is required by the language, stress on the appropriate syllable of the word, phrasing and pausing in connected speech, and intonation appropriate to the meaning of the communication, all add to the intelligibility of the speaker.

The *phonetic method* is an essential teaching aid for the child with a hearing problem. This method is an accurate means of representing visually the sound structure of the language. The procedure includes analysis of the articulation of the vowels, diphthongs, and consonants of the language. It also includes analysis of lengthening of sound, stress on syllables of words, stress on words in groups, phrasing, intonation, and their visual representation. Furthermore, the phonetic approach to language provides opportunities for auditory training so necessary for the child with a hearing loss.

The phonetic method is combined with other aspects of language learning: *vocabulary building, reading, writing,* and other *visual aids.* Since the child's eyes will have to substitute for much of the work of his ears, colorful and varied visual aids are necessary prerequisites for the education of this child. In working with the young hypacusic child, the therapist should provide practice in all the elements of spoken language. This is accomplished by using materials and vocabulary appropriate to the age of the youngster. It is important to provide a variety of material and activity. When a word is introduced, a picture should be used to illustrate the meaning. Pantomime may also be employed when a picture is not useful. These visual aids must always be accompanied by saying the word.

To accompany this direct teaching of the sound structure of the language, there should be enjoyment of the speech arts and of music. Choral speaking, creative dramatics, improvisations, story telling, and singing will afford practice in the phonetic elements of spoken language.

The speech therapist should familiarize herself not only with the child's medical history, but with his emotional and intellectual background as well. This knowledge will help immeasurably in applying the methods of speech instruction already suggested. It should be remembered that in comparison with knowledge of physical growth, one usually knows less about emotional development. It may be said that there is unquestionably an ordered emotional maturation just as there is an ordered intellectual and physical development. Unfortunately, there are no standardized tests for determining the normality of the emotional development of the child.

West (4) mentions, in connection with correction of speech defects, a quality which he calls "residual diathesis" or the "X factor." This entity comprises the child's ability to overcome difficulties. It may also include his personal potential for adjustment and improvement in spite of his defect. The speech clinician may tap this source for therapy after observation of the child's potential.

Group work in addition to individualized therapy, is usually more successful than exclusively individual instruction. The use of three-dimensional objects, bright and large pictures and other visual aids, are of great importance in the teaching program of the hypacusic child. Benefits also result from participation in arts and crafts.

CENTRAL AUDITORY PATHOLOGY

In connection with word deafness, Kastein and Fowler (5) state that some children found in schools for the deaf are diagnosed as cases of peripheral deafness, but do not "fit the picture of the deaf child." They do not respond to the training received by the hard of hearing. Kastein reports on a special study of the language development of these children made at Columbia-Presbyterian Medical Center in New York.

The assumption upon which Kastein's study was based is that development of language consists of several functions which evolve as a result of interdependent progression in the child, parallel with the maturation of his central nervous system. These functions consist of peripheral sense perception, mental concepts (precepts), symbolic behavior, psychomotor functions, figure-ground discrimination, intelligence, and emotional adjustment. This basic assumption is also stated by West (4) in his description of normal development of speech and language in the child.

Many conditions were found to cause delayed language development in the Kastein study. Anacusis, hypacusis, dysacusis, expressive language disorders, mental retardation as well as other deficits of the central nervous system, and emotional disorders were all found responsible. Kastein states that contrary to the child with peripheral auditory impairment, the child who is dysacusic (word deaf) cannot use compensatory mechanisms such as gestures. He is, therefore, much more handicapped than the peripherally deaf child.

Many conclusions have been drawn as a result of the Kastein study. A lack or deviation in language and speech development in children with word deafness is often the first and only manifestation of a central nervous system deficit. The earlier the diagnosis is made, the more precisely the areas of impairment can be detected. The earlier the training is started, the better the chances of habilitation. The child's intelligence plays a special role since the language-impaired youngster requires more than average intelligence to overcome his handicap. Even after prolonged training, dysacusic children may still have learning problems and difficulties in abstract thinking.

Psychomotor training coupled with reading and writing at an early age yield good results in the habilitation of the child with language impairment. Parent counseling and a home training program are essential in the habilitation of these children.

THERAPEUTIC SUGGESTIONS FOR PARENTS

Prolonged listening can be fatiguing. It is, therefore, wise to vary or reinforce auditory stimuli with appeals to the other senses. It is important for parents to provide many opportunities for listening in the home. These may be in the form of reading or telling stories, listening to recordings appropriate to the age of the listener, or listening to carefully selected television or radio programs. Above all, listening to and reacting to conversation in the home stimulates comprehension and production of language on the part of the child. Listening must be active to be valuable in language development in the child. The outcome of listening should be action either in the form of stimulated thought or in the form of response through speech.

Speech therapists should work closely with parents of children who have hearing problems. It is essential to the success of the speech program, that the parents cooperate by continuing speech training in the home. The following suggestions to parents are helpful:

1. Continue talking to the child as though he had normal hearing. Unfortunately, there is a tendency to stop talking to a hearing handicapped child. Avoid this.

2. Do not expect the child to reply when speaking to him.

3. Do not expect the child to repeat words after they are spoken by others. The youngster may attempt to say a word or two. This must come voluntarily as it does with children who possess normal hearing acuity.

4. Parents should respond whenever the child is speaking to them.

5. Parents should be sure that adequate light is provided when addressing the child. Light should not shine in the child's eyes.

6. Always attempt to *show* the child what is being talked about, either by holding up the object or a picture of it. Pictures should be simple and life-like, with clear outlines. Avoid fantastic pictures or cartoons.

7. Speak to the child in simple, grammatically correct, complete sentences. Repeat the same sentence at a definite time of day or in a certain place. Sentences such as, "This is your coat. Put on your coat," are helpful.

8. Teach the child rhythms by dancing to music or by waving the hands in time with the music.

9. The parent should keep her/his face on a level with that of the child when addressing him. One should sit in a low chair when speaking.

10. Speak naturally. Neither drawl, whisper, nor exaggerate lip movements.

11. Avoid gestures while talking. The child will not look at the speaker's mouth if gestures are being used. Furthermore, never indicate by a gesture what may be explained by demonstrating the object.

In general, parents should be reminded to "pour out" speech to the child with a hearing disability. Since the youngster lives in a speaking world, he must become used to comprehending thought through visual cues and with the help of a hearing aid if one is indicated. Since the home environment has a lasting influence on the deaf child's emotional and intellectual growth, the parents should be taught to perform an integral part in the language and speech development of this child.

Furthermore, increased symbolization and comprehension through looking at, and listening to language will help the child's reasoning powers and his own production of both written and spoken language. For as Karlin has stated, "Poverty of language in the hypacusic child impairs his ability to think."

REFERENCES

(1) Best, C. H., and Taylor, N. B.: *The Physiological Basis of Medical Practice.* 7th Edition. Baltimore, The Williams & Wilkins Co., 1961.
(2) West, R.: Personal Communication to the Authors.
(3) Luriya, A. R., and Yudovich, F. Y.: *Speech and the Development of Mental Processes in the Child.* London, Staples Press, 1959.
(4) West, R., Ansberry, M., and Carr, A.: *The Rehabilitation of Speech.* New York, Harper & Brothers, 1957.
(5) Kastein, S., and Fowler, E. P., Jr.: Differential Diagnosis of Communication Disorders in Children Referred for Hearing Tests. *Arch. Otolaryng., 60:*468, October, 1954.

Chapter 13

CLEFT PALATE AND CLEFT LIP

INTRODUCTION

Congenital cleft palate and cleft lip denote a partial or a complete failure of union in early embryonic life between the separate processes which form the lips, alveolar border and hard and soft palates. Figures 39 and 40 illustrate varieties of un-operated clefts of the lip and palate. Involvement may vary from a fissure of the uvula to a complete division of the structures anterior to it. The disunion may be confined to the soft palate alone or it may affect the hard palate. Occasionally, the lip is involved without a deformity of the hard or soft palates. Fogh-Anderson (1) states that the prevalence of cleft lip and cleft palate is approximately 1 per 1000 births. Schwartz (2) finds the condition to occur more frequently in boys than in girls. It is more common in members of the white race.

ETIOLOGY

The cause of the condition is not definitely known. Present consensus supports the thought that more than one factor may play an etiologic role. Studies on identical and non-identical twins indicate that genetic factors may be one of the causes. Fogh-Anderson investigated the distribution of cleft palate and cleft lip in Denmark. He demonstrated a familial history in thirty per cent of the families of 903 patients seen by him. Thus, the condition tends to occur in successive generations and in siblings. Maternal malnutrition has also been suggested as an etiologic factor. Experimentally, cleft palate has been produced by maternal nutritional deficiencies in strains of animals ordinarily free of this anomaly. Cleft palate and cleft lip are occasionally accompanied by structural deformities in other parts of the body involving the skeletal system, the nervous system, and the diges-

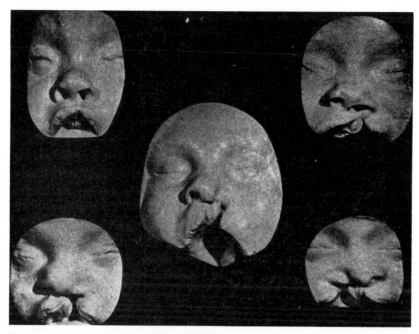

Figure 39. Casts of the upper lip and nose in infants with several varieties of unoperated unilateral clefts of the lip. From Samuel Pruzansky's Description, Classification, and Analysis of Unoperated Clefts of the Lip and Palate, *American Journal of Orthodontics*, 39:590, 1953. Courtesy of C. V. Mosby Co., St. Louis, Missouri.

tive system. Thus, it may be found in conjunction with spina bifida, hydrocephalus, and imperforate anus.

On the basis of available embryological and histological evidence, it would appear that the noxious factors involved must manifest themselves between the sixth and tenth weeks of pregnancy. Normally, at about the fourth week of intrauterine life, an opening develops at the anterior end of the embryo which is known as the *stomodeum.* Five processes surround this opening: a single *frontonasal process,* two *maxillary processes,* and two *mandibular processes* (see Figure 41).

The time of union for these various structures is between the sixth to tenth weeks of intrauterine life. Once this time has passed and union has not taken place, the defect remains and the child is born with a malformation. Thus, it is evident that

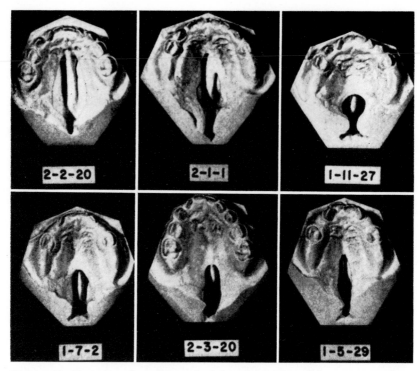

Figure 40. Varieties of unoperated cleft palate. The cleft may extend, in varying degrees, as far forward as the nasopalatine foramen. From Samuel Pruzansky's Description, Classification, and Anaylsis of Unoperated Clefts of the Lip and Palate, *American Journal of Orthodontics*, 39:590, 1953. Courtesy of C. V. Mosby Co., St. Louis, Missouri.

whatever the cause of the arrested development, this must occur during the first three months of pregnancy and most probably during the second month. Mothers will frequently tell the physician that they had a shock or some illness during the latter part of pregnancy. However, from embryologic studies, this could not have had an effect upon the development of cleft palate or cleft lip.

CLASSIFICATION

The classification of congenital cleft palate and cleft lip is not a universal one. Most classifications that appear in the literature are not completely descriptive. They frequently reflect the

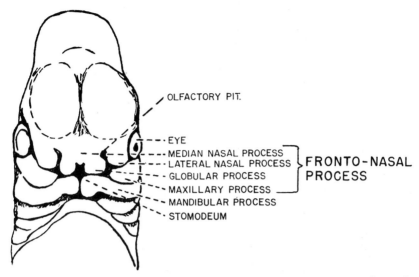

Figure 41. Formation of the face in a human embryo of the sixth week. From Muriel E. Morley's *Cleft Palate and Speech*, 5th Ed., 1962. Courtesy of E. & S. Livingstone Ltd., Edinburgh, Scotland.

clinical interest of a single professional group. The noted surgeon, Vilray P. Blair (3), in commenting on a classification of congenital clefts based on the surgical requirements, rather than on the anatomical differences, stated quite succinctly, "The surgery is shifting and the anatomy is fixed."

In accordance with the facts of the embryology, anatomy, and physiology of the cleft defect, Pruzansky (4), using the alveolar process as a focal point, divides the varieties of clefts of the palate and lip into four general categories. The alveolar process is that part of the maxillary process which forms the teeth ridge.

1. Those involving the lip alone (prealveolar).
2. Those involving the lip and palate (alveolar).
3. Those in which the palate alone is affected (postalveolar).
4. Congenital insufficiency of the palate.

Clefts of the Lip

The malformation may be complete, extending from the vermilion border of the lip to the floor of the nose, or it may be incomplete. Minimal defects involving only the vermilion border are observed, too. The defect may be unilateral (left or right), bilateral, or median (see Figure 39, page 241). The alveolar process, however, is intact.

Cleft Palate and Cleft Lip

In these cases, the alveolar process is *not* complete and forms the cleft. The cleft follows incisor sutures through the alveolus. Clefts of the palate and lip may be unilateral or bilateral. They may be complete or incomplete. In a complete unilateral cleft of the palate and lip, a direct communication exists between the oral and nasal cavities on that side of the palate in which the cleft is situated. The bilateral cleft palate and cleft lip may also be complete or incomplete. If incomplete, it may be symmetrical or asymmetrical, depending on the equality of involvement on both sides. Thus, a remarkable range of variation can be present in each category.

Cleft Palate

The alveolar process is complete and, therefore, neither the lip nor the alveolar process is involved. There may be bifid uvula, a cleft of only the soft palate or a cleft of both the soft palate and the hard palate. A cleft of the hard palate never occurs alone (see Figure 40, page 242).

Congenital Insufficiency of the Palate

Pruzansky (4) states that cleft palate is the kind of defect that can be "seen, felt, and heard." Congenital insufficiency of the palate, however, until recently, has been more readily heard than seen or felt. This anomaly is seldom apparent at birth. The first awareness of the defect occurs when the child develops the hypernasality characteristic of cleft palate speech.

The term *palatal insufficiency* is more descriptive of a physiological deficiency than of an anatomical defect. In reviewing the morphological variants that might contribute to inadequate velopharyngeal function, Dorrance (5) recognizes a number of factors. He points out that the velum (soft palate) might be too short or that the hard palate could be deficient in its antero-posterior dimensions. In others, both the hard and soft palates might be shorter than normal. Submucous clefts in the median line of the palatal processes, in the palatal aponeurosis, and in the muscles of the velum are often described in cases with congenital palatal insufficiency. In this condition, there is impaired movement of the palate without obvious signs of arrest in development.

ANATOMICAL AND PHYSIOLOGICAL MECHANISM

The palate forms the roof of the mouth and separates the oral from the nasal cavities. It consists of two parts, the hard palate anteriorly and the soft palate posteriorly.

The soft palate is capable of fine and rapid movements essential for good speech. It separates the nasal cavities from the pharynx and mouth during the act of swallowing and during speech, except for the production of the nasal sounds *m, n,* and *ng.* In this case, the oral exit is closed by the lips or tongue and the sound waves pass behind the soft palate and out through the nasopharynx and nostrils.

To prevent the air stream from passing into the nose, it is essential that there should be in the nasopharynx, some means of completely shutting off the nasal cavities. The closure is achieved predominantly by the synchronous action of two muscles, the *superior constrictor* of the pharynx and the *levator palati.* These muscles, acting together, form the *palatopharyngeal sphincter* which, when closed, prevents the passage of air from the pharynx into the nose (see Figure 42). This action is necessary to voice all non-nasal sounds.

Wardill and Whillis (6) describe the physiologic nasopharyngeal closure by observing the action of the two muscles primarily involved. The levator palati arises from the temporal bone at the base of the skull and enters the soft palate on each side of the central line. The soft palate is raised in preparation for speech by the contraction of this muscle into a position almost in contact with the posterior wall of the pharynx, the muscles of which have also contracted, causing bunching of the mucosa in the lateral walls to form *Passavant's cushion* (see Figures 11, 12, page 56). Morley (7) states that the inward movement of the posterior

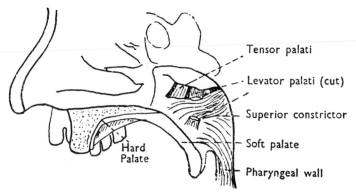

Figure 42. Dissection of the normal nasopharynx (Wardill). From Muriel E. Morley's *Cleft Palate and Speech*, 5th Ed., 1962. Courtesy of E. & S. Livingstone Ltd., Edinburgh, Scotland.

and lateral walls of the pharynx is as important for pharyngeal closure as the upward and backward movement of the soft palate. Finally, the superior constrictor of the pharynx maintains its contractile state as long as speech is produced, thus keeping the ridge of Passavant raised and causing narrowing of the naso-pharynx from side to side. The superior constrictor of the pharynx is a complex muscle in the wall of the pharynx, some fibers of which pass into the soft palate.

Thus, velopharyngeal closure is produced by the upward and backward movement of the soft palate, coincident with a sphinc-ter-like action at the lowest part of the nasopharynx, shutting off the nasopharynx. During deglutition and during phonation, ex-cept for the sounds *m, n,* and *ng,* the soft palate elevates, making contact with the posterior and lateral walls of the pharynx. The complicated synergies that contribute to this multidimensional contraction serve to separate the nasopharynx from the oro-pharynx.

This mechanism of velopharyngeal closure can be studied by cephalometric roentgenography. It has been observed that the soft palate is raised higher for some sounds than for others. It is raised more for *k* than for *t* and higher for *oo* and *ee* than for *ah.* It is also higher for voiced than for unvoiced consonants. During blowing, the palate rises to its maximum height. In cleft palate, this velopharyngeal closure cannot be achieved. Deglutition is impaired and in phonation, the air stream is misdirected through the nose.

Cleft palate and cleft lip disturb the functions of sucking, mastication, deglutition, respiration, Eustachian ventilation, and speech.

NATURE OF CLEFT PALATE SPEECH

Speech defects resulting from cleft palate and cleft lip are characterized by distortions of many sounds, serious hypernasality, substitution of laryngeal and pharyngeal sounds and nasal snorts for speech sounds ordinarily produced in the mouth. There is generalized emission of air through the nose during speech.

Hearing loss is commonly associated with cleft palate due to the interference with Eustachian physiology and subsequent middle ear infection. Such hearing deficit imposes further handicaps upon speech, since speech reception and speech discrimination are limited.

The speech and hearing disabilities associated with cleft palate and cleft lip frequently act as deterrents to school progress, induce extensive personality changes in the patient, and interfere with satisfactory social and vocational adjustment. The cosmetic defects of the nose and lip may also reinforce and encourage inappropriate personality development.

It can be said that with any degree of cleft palate, preventing separation of the oral from the nasal cavity, normal speech is impossible. The requisite air pressure in the mouth for the production of any explosive consonant is unobtainable. Cleft palate speech is due to the fact that in articulation of nearly all consonants, air which should be expelled through the mouth escapes through the cleft into the nose. The production of all consonants, except the nasal *m*, *n*, and *ng*, is defective. This diversion of air into the nose results in an unpleasant nasal quality to speech. It causes a hollow voice quality with weak production of those sounds which require the building up of air pressure within the mouth. The child tries to limit the escape of air through the nose by contracting the nostrils. This is effected by raising the upper lip and compressing the nostrils. These muscular efforts produce facial contortions and grimaces.

Distortions of Speech Sounds

There are two main reasons for distortions of sounds in cleft palate speech. First, air cannot be held within the oral cavity as a result of malformation of the palate. It is deflected into the nasal passages. Second, anomalies of the articulators, especially the lips, teeth, alveolar ridge, and soft palate cause severe articulatory distortions. Furthermore, some children with cleft palate and cleft lip show a loss in hearing. Because of this additional auditory handicap, they cannot articulate sounds properly, since they are not able to hear them.

The vowel sounds have a nasal timbre in cleft palate speech. The disturbed vowel quality is one of the most conspicuous features of a child with cleft palate. The vowels most affected are those in which the soft palate is most strongly contracted, namely, *oo*(u) and *ee*(i).

Koepp-Baker (8) observes that the plosive sounds are commonly absent, weak, or distorted. If the palate is open and no obturation by a speech-aid is present, it is impossible to achieve the necessary air pressure within the oral cavity for the plosive phase of consonant production. In severe cases where the defect has not been treated, the patient strains in an effort to articulate. The result is that the vocal cords close sharply and then open quickly to release air. This action produces the *glottal stop* which replaces many of the plosive consonants *p, b, t, d, k,* and *g*. The glottal stop may also be used by children with cleft palate for other consonant sounds. This action imposes a strain upon the larynx. For this reason, the child is often hoarse. Even after surgical repair, nasal speech together with weak speech qualities may remain, if steps are not taken to train the muscles of the palate and throat. The muscles of the throat will be developed by the therapeutic speech program to be discussed later.

Koepp-Baker (8) states that the fricatives, in cleft plate speech, are either absent or suffer distortion because of the substitution of characteristic pharyngeal fricatives or the improper posture-movement sequences. The loss of air pressure by leakage into the nasopharynx and nose during the production of fricatives is very apparent in cleft palate speech at normal and rapid rates. The voiceless fricatives are frequently voiced because of stress or effort of production. Furthermore, when the child tries to produce the *s* sound, the air is misdirected through the nose with a hissing or snorting quality.

Another factor in the production of nasality, apart from the abnormal patency of the connection between the oropharynx and nasopharynx, is the role of the tongue and mandible. Some investigators believe that at least some of the nasality of cleft palate patients results from the persistent habit of elevating the mandible and dorsum of the tongue during speech. This movement has two possible ill effects. First, it reduces the size of the opening into the oral cavity. Second, it tends to divide the combined oral and pharyngeal cavities into two markedly disproportionate cavities producing a resonance which acoustically one calls nasality. This tendency for cleft palate patients to hold the dorsum of the tongue high makes it impossible for them to use the tip of the tongue, which is necessary for the accurate production of many speech sounds.

There are other anatomical factors, besides the cleft itself, which play a role in the production of cleft palate speech. An important secondary cause of defective speech is the irregular shape of the mouth. Furthermore, in a series of measurements of normal and cleft palate skulls, Wardill (9) demonstrates that in the cleft palate skulls, the dimensions of the pharynx are increased in the antero-posterior direction and from side to side. The increase in width is found to be greater than the increase in the antero-posterior diameter. This increase in the size of the nasopharynx will produce the well known cleft palate type of speech. To reduce the increased dimension of the nasopharynx, the operation of pharyngeoplasty was devised in conjunction with the various types of operations for closure of the cleft.

EXAMINATION AND DIAGNOSIS

The conditions of cleft palate and cleft lip present few diagnostic problems, with the exception of congenital insufficiency of the palate. Koepp-Baker (10) states that direct visual and digital examinations of the lip, the nasal, oral, and pharyngeal spaces and structures, together with a careful phonetic study, provide adequate facts for differential diagnosis of the deformity. Complete otological and audiological examinations are important. Thorough orthodontic examination adds indispensable information for treatment planning. A general pediatric examination is indicated for evaluation of physical and mental health as well as for the possible discovery of associated congenital abnormalities.

Pediatric Conditions Associated with Cleft Palate

Micrognathia, or hypoplasia of the mandible, is a rare congenital anomaly. When the hypoplasia is marked, the tongue may be displaced posteriorly, the condition being known as *glossoptosis.* Glossoptosis results in inadequate respiratory exchange and cyanosis. If cleft palate is associated with the micrognathia and glossoptosis, the condition is called the *Pierre Robin Syndrome.* Here, the respiratory distress may be pronounced and *glossopexy* may be necessary as a life-saving procedure.

TREATMENT OF CLEFT PALATE AND CLEFT LIP

The treatment of cleft palate and cleft lip requires the cooperation of the plastic surgeon, the dental surgeon (especially the orthodontist), the speech therapist, social workers, and others. In spite of the fact that the ideal objective in cleft palate surgery is to obviate the need for speech therapy, until that day arrives one should enlist the aid of a speech clinician.

To make it possible for a cleft palate child to acquire normal speech, he must be provided with the means to separate the oral from the nasal cavities. Treatment *usually* requires surgery, orthodontic treatment, speech therapy, and social readjustment. It *may* require the use of an obturator. One or all of these treatments may have to be employed.

One must consider the most opportune time at which the operations for cleft lip and cleft palate should be performed. Most authorities agree that it is good surgical practice to repair cleft lip soon after birth, within the first three weeks to three months of life. It is important to establish early muscular function of the lips to reduce feeding problems at an early age.

Palatal surgery is usually deferred until a later date, although there is much less unanimity of opinion concerning time of palatal surgery as contrasted to lip surgery. Many plastic surgeons believe that palatal closure should be performed between eighteen months to twenty-four months following birth. From the special viewpoint of adequate speech development, early operative intervention is advisable before defective speech habits become well established. Some surgeons, however, postpone operation to close the palatal vault until well after infancy to allow for maxillary growth. Ricketts (11) studied the head development of normal children and of those having palatal or lip defects. His findings led him to suggest that if these structures are not interfered with by early surgery, the general growth of the mouth and head follows a more normal pattern.

An obturator may be used in cases where surgery cannot be performed such as in extremely large clefts, cases of repeated surgical failures, and in poor operative risks. The obturator is a prosthetic device similar to a dental plate which is worn by the child to form a roof to the mouth and cover the cleft (see Figure 43). The obturator assists articulation. It can also be used post-

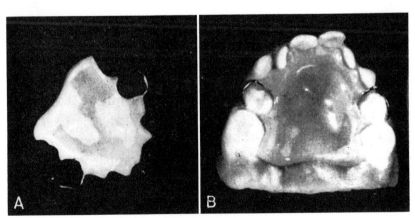

Figure 43. The obturator, or dental plate, used to cover a fistula in the palate.

    A. The Appliance.

    B. The Appliance *in situ.*

From Muriel E. Morley's *Cleft Palate and Speech,* 5th Ed., 1962. Courtesy of E. & S. Livingstone Ltd., Edinburgh, Scotland.

operatively. The obturator, which often has a bulb attachment, becomes a speech aid and can be worn by the child at the age of deciduous dentition. It has been used in children as young as two and one-half years of age.

Morley (7) is of the opinion that operation in infancy for repair of the palate offers the best prognosis. She states that three factors have to be considered when deciding the best age for operation. The optimal time will be governed by the mortality rate, orofacial development as exhibited by maxillary growth, and speech development. From a consideration of all these factors, Morley states that operation during infancy is desirable since present day methods of surgery render unlikely the danger to life. Second, operation will not necessarily interfere with palatal growth. Furthermore, she believes that early operative intervention will provide the requisite conditions for the natural spontaneous development of speech before poor speaking habits have had a chance to become deeply rooted.

A description of the various surgical techniques in cleft palate surgery is of use mainly for the surgeon and is described fully in plastic surgical textbooks and papers. Suffice it to say that operative methods have been developed along the three following lines:

1. Closure of the cleft by median suture.

2. Flap methods in which a flap of tissue is used to close the cleft.

3. Methods involving orthodontic mobilization of the palatal halves prior to surgical closure.

The aim of surgery is not merely to close the cleft, but to restore the physiological function to the palate once velopharyngeal closure has been achieved. The production of good speech is the criterion by which the operative procedure is judged.

The removal of adenoids and tonsils can aggravate the speech defect in children with cleft palate. The adenoids are situated on the posterior wall of the pharynx. When they are removed, the soft palate must now span a greater distance during its elevation, in order to contact the posterior pharyngeal wall and effect closure between the oral and nasal cavities. In some cases, however, if enlarged tonsils and adenoids produce a conductive hearing defect via encroachment on the Eustachian tube, it may be necessary to remove them to prevent further hearing loss.

Surgery is usually the procedure of choice in closing the cleft, except in cases in which the cleft is extremely large or in cases where repeated operative intervention has led to poor tissue with which to work. Koepp-Baker (12) states that surgical closure of the palate and velum is not always a wise procedure if the goal of improved speech is to be obtained. When palates of inadequate tissue substance have been closed, the velopharyngeal mechanism is at a functional disadvantage. Furthermore, late prosthetic treatment of these children is often made more difficult.

SPEECH THERAPY

Speech therapy should follow surgery and should not precede it. The child may become discouraged if he attempts to correct his faults at a time when he has little possibility of achieving good results.

The following factors govern the eventual outcome of speech training:

1. Anatomical and physiological results of surgery, orthodontia, and prosthetic devices.
2. The intelligence of the child.
3. The acuity of hearing.
4. The level and type of speech development at the time of operation.
5. The age at which speech therapy commences.
6. The personality of the child and the environment in which he lives.

The question is often asked as to whether group speech therapy or individual therapy is best for the child. A combination of both is at times highly desirable. Exercises for the soft palate and the development of correct habits of breath direction are frequently more enjoyable when performed in the company of other children. The child finds himself no longer alone, but in company with others who have a similar or even a more pronounced speech defect. However, a certain amount of individual training is imperative. The child must have individual ear training to make possible the recognition of the difference between correct and faulty speech sounds.

Morley (7) has divided speech therapy for cleft palate into four groups, each group having appropriate exercises for the development of correct speaking habits.

First, the child should be given training in correct breath direction. This involves the use of both palatal and pharyngeal muscles to produce closure of the palatopharyngeal sphincter, dividing the oral from the nasal cavities.

Second, coordination of the palatal and pharyngeal muscles with the articulatory muscles of the tongue and lips should be practiced.

Third, instruction in correct articulation of each vowel and consonant sound and the ability to use each sound in combination to form syllables, words, and finally sentences at the speed necessary for incorporation into fluent speech should be provided. This also includes ear training exercises.

Fourth, the child must learn to introduce these sounds into speech, entailing the unconscious use of new and correct habits of articulation.

Cleft palate speech has been generally regarded as a very resistant form of speech disability. Koepp-Baker (8) states that this has been largely due to the former stress on the part of most speech clinicians on the phonatory aspects of cleft palate. Today, emphasis is placed on finding ways of improving the articulation of the child with cleft palate.

The dictum that "speaking is learned by speaking" applies especially to the child with cleft palate. Koepp-Baker (8) states that it is now generally agreed that the initial attack on cleft palate speech should be made upon the defects in articulation. Malarticulation is attacked by training with correct syllable formation. Many speech clinicians combine the anterior plosives with low vowels and proceed to the fricatives with low and mid-vowels. Syllables with high-vowel cores are apt to be the most resistant. This training which involves revision of habitual tongue position will improve resonance and voice production. The result will be the greatest and most immediate change in the intelligibility of speech and the quality of voice.

REFERENCES

(1) Fogh-Anderson, P.: *Inheritance of Harelip and Cleft Palate.* Copenhagen, Nyt Nordisk Forlag, Arnold Busck, 1942.

(2) Schwartz, R.: Familial Incidence of Cleft Palate. *J. Speech & Hearing Disorders, 19*:2, 1954.

(3) Blair, V. P.: Discussion of Davis, J. S., and Ritchie, H. P.: Classification of Congential Clefts of the Lip and Palate. *J. A. M. A.,* 79:1323, October 14, 1922.

(4) Pruzansky, S.: Description, Classification, and Analysis of Unoperated Clefts of the Lip and Palate. *Am. J. Orthodontics, 39*: No. 8, 590, August, 1953.

(5) Dorrance, G. M.: *The Operative Story of Cleft Palate.* Philadelphia, W. B. Saunders Co., 1933.

(6) Wardill, W. E. M., and Whillis, J.: Movements of the Soft Palate. *Surg. Gynec. & Obstet., 62*:836, 1936.

(7) Morley, M. E.: *Cleft Palate and Speech.* Edinburgh & London, E. & S. Livingstone Ltd., 1962.

(8) Koepp-Baker, H.: Speech Problems of the Person with Cleft Palate and Cleft Lip. In, Travis, L. E.: *Handbook of Speech Pathology.* New York, Appleton-Century-Crofts, 1957.

(9) Wardill, W. E. M.: Cleft Palate. *Brit. J. Surg., 26*:61, 1928.

(10) Koepp-Baker, H.: *The Rehabilitation of the Person with Cleft Lip and Cleft Palate.* Prepared for the National Society for Crippled Children and Adults, Inc., the American Speech and Hearing Association, and the New York University College of Medicine—American Medical Association Scientific Exhibit, Atlantic City, June 6-10, 1949.

(11) Ricketts, R. M.: The Significance of Variation in the Cranial Base and Soft Structures. Newsletter, *Am. Assoc. Cleft Palate Rehab., 3*:5, 1952.

(12) Koepp-Baker, H.: Pathomorphology of Cleft Palate and Cleft Lip. In, Travis, L. E.: *Handbook of Speech Pathology.* New York, Appleton-Century-Crofts, 1957.

Chapter 14

CEREBRAL PALSY

CEREBRAL palsy is a neuromuscular disorder that has been known for some time. Little (1), an English orthopedic surgeon, first described the condition in 1862. It remained for Phelps (2), however, in 1936, to coin the term cerebral palsy. The word *cerebral* indicates a condition related to the head. The word *palsy* refers to a disturbance of the muscles or joints. Thus, cerebral palsy is a condition in which a number of neuromuscular abnormalities result from damage to the brain at an early stage of development.

The incidence of cerebral palsy births per year is purported by Phelps (3) in 1945 to be 7 for every 100,000 population. Although socio-economic status and geographic location do not appear to be factors, sex, race, and position of offspring in the family tree all seem to play a role. More boys than girls appear to have the condition. There seems to be a higher incidence of cerebral palsy in the white race. Finally, as Cardwell (4) points out, the first born appears to be more vulnerable to contracting cerebral palsy. Only rarely are two or more children in the same family afflicted.

ETIOLOGY

There are innumerable factors involved in the formation of the defects occurring in cerebral palsy. The causes may be divided into three categories. First, there are *prenatal* factors. Second, one must consider *paranatal* conditions. Third, *postnatal* conditions have been implicated as causative agents in the development of cerebral palsy.

It was formerly thought that, in most cases, cerebral palsy was due to mechanical injury arising out of trauma during the birth process. Recent literature indicates that mechanical birth injury is not quite as common a causal agent as was originally thought. Today, more significance is attached to hazards occur-

256

ring in early states of embryonic development and to problems of oxygen deprivation which may occur at any time before, during, or after birth.

Infectious and metabolic diseases are high on the list of prenatal causes of cerebral palsy. Toxoplasmosis, severe anemia, and German measles are frequent causes. Cerebral anoxia resulting from erythroblastosis fetalis is one of the common causes of brain injury.

Mechanical factors constitute the majority of the paranatal causes of cerebral palsy. Paranatal causes are those conditions that result directly from the process of birth delivery. Subdural hemorrhage occurring as a result of ruptures from delicate blood vessels of the brain or of meninges comprises the most common of the paranatal causes. The result of sudden changes in pressure on the extremely friable vascular system of the premature infant is numbered among other paranatal etiologic factors.

Cardwell (4) states that postnatal factors contribute about ten per cent of all cases of cerebral palsy. Among the most common postnatal causes are mechanical injury, circulatory defects, infectious diseases such as whooping cough and scarlet fever, toxic states, and neoplasms.

TYPES OF CEREBRAL PALSY

Orthopedics, neurology, and physical medicine and rehabilitation classify cerebral palsy into various groups according to the criteria of type, location, and severity.

The type of cerebral palsy indicates the kind of neuromuscular involvement and can be divided into the following: *athetoid, spastic, ataxic, tremor,* and *rigidity.*

Injury to the basal ganglia, whether it be a lesion or necrosis due to cerebral anoxia, produces *athetosis.* Athetosis is characterized by a twisting, serpentine series of involuntary muscular movements, progressing from proximal to distal areas and arriving in waves following each other. *Spasticity* results from damage to the motor cortex located in the precentral gyrus or in the pyramidal pathways. It is characterized by increased muscular tension preventing the normal rhythmic flow of movement. *Ataxia* is usually the result of cerebellar dysfunction although it may also be caused to a lesser extent by lesions located in the vestibular portion of the eighth cranial nerve. Ataxic individuals exhibit loss of control, balance, and space orientation. *Tremor,* like athetosis, is caused by a lesion in the basal ganglia. It is characterized by involuntary rhythmic movements. It differs from athetosis in that the movements are regular and rhythmic. *Rigidity* is somewhat similar to spasticity and is due to widespread involvement of the basal ganglia and cerebral cortex. Lastly, there may be multiple combinations involving one or more of the above disorders. Thus, both spasticity and athetosis may be found together in the same child.

A second classification of cerebral palsy is based on the location of the neuromuscular involvement. Thus, one uses the terms *monoplegia, paraplegia, triplegia, quadriplegia,* or right and left *hemiplegia* depending upon the number of extremities involved or the side of the body affected. Although speech pathology may be present in any one of the above mentioned paralyses, speech dysfunction is least likely to occur where monoplegia or paraplegia are involved.

The degree of severity of the neuromuscular involvement serves as a useful guide for prognosis and the ultimate results of therapeutic regimens. Thus, the terms mild, moderate, and severe, when applied to the neuromuscular damage in the cerebral-palsied child, will give some indication of what results might be expected through the various programs of physical medicine and rehabilitation.

SYMPTOMS AND SIGNS

The cerebral-palsied child exhibits various deficiencies in normal growth and development as a result of neuromuscular imbalance emanating from cerebral pathology. Many of these sensory and motor abnormalities have a direct bearing on the acquisition of meaningful speech and language.

Hopkins, Bice, and Colton (5) show that children with cerebral palsy have a high incidence of visual and hearing impairment. Obviously, those children with the greatest loss of vision and hearing will be less able to learn proper speech habits. Perceptual disturbances in the visual, auditory, and kinesthetic fields are also found in cerebral-palsied individuals and present barriers to the development of oral and written communication.

The onset of sitting, crawling, standing, and walking is delayed in cases of cerebral palsy. Speech is also impaired as a result of general delay in motor development.

Investigators demonstrate some correlation between early intellectual ability and the development of speech. Many studies have been done comparing the I.Q.s of the cerebral-palsied child with that of the normal. In general, a majority of children with cerebral palsy have I.Q.s considerably below average. There is even a large per cent who are so seriously intellectually retarded that they may be classified as mentally defective. Naturally, as was shown in an earlier chapter, severe mental retardation has a very adverse influence on the development of speech.

Hearing Disability

The loss of hearing found in the child with CP (cerebral palsy) can be a tremendous impediment to the normal acquisition of speech. The incidence of hearing loss varies considerably from one investigator to the other. Rutherford (6) gives as high an incidence as forty-one per cent while Hopkins, Bice, and Colton (5) quote a figure of five per cent. Differences in the incidence of hearing loss in cerebral palsy result from lack of standardization of the reference points for hearing loss, methods of testing, and perhaps population sampling.

Considerable attention has been focused on the higher incidence of hearing loss in athetoids. The Rh negative factor is a possible cause of certain types of hearing loss. Hardy (7) states that the highest number of auditory problems develop in the athetoid type. The exact anatomical location of the lesion in the "Rh deaf" child is still a matter of conjecture. Saltzman (8) believes the lesion to be in the basal ganglia rather than in the acoustic nerve or ear itself. Goodhill (9) states that the defect may be in the auditory nuclei of the brain stem or in the midbrain.

There is also the problem of whether the Rh child with a hearing loss has actually sustained damage to the auditory apparatus or whether he is "aphasic." This problem was discussed in a symposium at the 1955 Convention of the American Speech and Hearing Association. The various reports cited indicate that the question still exists regarding central vs. peripheral hearing involvement in the Rh athetoid child. Mecham, Berko, and Berko (10), in a summary of experimental evidence on this subject state that, "Although many of the children may be peripherally hard of hearing or deaf, a great number probably have involvement of the auditory pathways on a neurological level higher than the cochlea or acoustic nerve and that many of them manifest aphasic-like language problems."

Psychological Disturbances

The child with cerebral palsy has many psychological problems that tend to retard growth and development of language. Although injury involving the motor areas of the brain is the cardinal abnormality in cerebral palsy, the tendency toward increased emotional lability and easy distractibility are consequences that have a direct influence on speech development. The emotionally disturbed child frequently makes a poor adjustment to his environment. If there is lack of motivation for the attainment of adequate speech and language in the environment, there is frequently lack of responsiveness to even the best of therapeutic and educational regimens.

Perseveration is a factor to be considered in children with cerebral palsy. The CP (cerebral palsy) child has a tendency to repeat previously rewarded responses, rather than to make adequate responses to the succeeding portions of a series of communicative interactions. In addition, previously learned activities do not become automatic as with the child having normal growth and development. Therefore, while the normal child may be rarely concerned with tongue placement or proper breathing during the course of speaking, the cerebral-palsied child frequently keeps these actions at a conscious level.

Thus, the emotional disturbances of the child with cerebral palsy, such as vasomotor lability, perseveration, hyperirritability, and attention disturbances all tend to retard the development of speech and language skills.

SPEECH DEFECTS IN CEREBRAL PALSY

Many different types of speech disorders are present in the child with cerebral palsy as a result of his multiple sensory, motor, and emotional problems. Although absolute figures differ, most investigators believe that approximately seventy per cent of children with cerebral palsy have some abnormality of speech and/or hearing.

In a discussion of language disorders in cerebral palsy, the question is often raised as to whether there is a characteristic "cerebral palsy speech." The speech of the cerebral palsied as a whole is slow, jerky, labored, and often unintelligible. Wepman (11) describes cerebral palsy speech as slow and scanning. West (12) describes visible features of the spastic which can be recognized. However, no acoustic differences are pointed out between the athetoid and the spastic. Berry and Eisenson (13) point to differences among athetoid, spastic, and ataxic cerebral-palsied speech as follows:

1. The athetoid presents articulatory problems that vary from complete mutism and dysarthria on one end of the scale to very slight articulatory disturbances on the other end. There are also phonetic changes as exhibited by whispered, hoarse, or ventricular phonation. The rhythmicity of breathing is also greatly disturbed.

2. Spastic speech possesses profound articulatory disturbances. Laryngeal muscle abnormalities lead to sudden, explosive increases in volume or rapid changes in pitch. Speech is labored, slow, and without vocal inflection.

3. The speech of the ataxic is recognized by a slurring of articulation which soon lapses into unintelligibility if speech is continued beyond phrases or short sentences. Rhythm is abnormal, and vocal pitch, loudness, and quality are monotonous or spasmodic.

Rutherford (14) believes that there is no characteristic speech that could be identified as being cerebral palsied. Mecham, Berko, and Berko (10) are of the opinion that, "Differences in the speech of the cerebral-palsied children and non-cerebral-palsied children are more apparent in degree than in quality."

They conclude by stating that cerebral palsy speech as a whole tends to be slow, irregular, effortful, and rather unintelligible. Such characteristics, they feel, comprise "cerebral palsy speech."

Many studies have been performed in an effort to determine the incidence of speech disorders in the various types of cerebral palsy. Although variability is present, probably due to differences in sampling, the majority of investigators state that the athetoid type has the largest incidence of speech defects.

DELAY IN DEVELOPMENT OF SPEECH

The developmental delay in the normal onset of speech must be discussed prior to a consideration of the individual speech defects. The variability of this factor is tremendous. One cerebral-palsied child may have a slight delay or no delay in the onset of speech. Another child may exhibit mutism as a result of complete lack of speech development. The factors influencing delay in speech are: emotional disturbances, hearing impairment, sensory and motor dysfunction, aphasia, and generalized intellectual retardation.

The neuromuscular handicaps of the cerebral-palsied child frequently make him unable to compete successfully with other children in the external environment. Emotional problems develop, especially in the form of anxiety, and the child may reject his external environment in an attempt to rid himself of noxious stimuli. Associations of individuals in the external environment are mediated through the use of language. Once the environment is rejected, the need for social intercourse may cease and language development may not be necessary. Consequent to lack of environmental interest, these children are often kept in a state of infantilism and therefore are not encouraged along the lines of growth and development.

There is a close relationship between hearing disability and delay in language development. This association should lead one to explore the possibility of a hearing loss when examining a child with cerebral palsy coupled with a speech impediment.

Cerebral palsy implies injury to brain tissue. Sensory and motor involvement can certainly contribute toward faulty speech development. Thus, lack of coordination of the articulators coupled with malfunction of the respiratory mechanism contribute greatly toward speech problems in cerebral palsy.

Many investigators believe aphasia to be a large contributory factor in speech disorders of the cerebral palsied. Both cerebral palsy and aphasia are products of brain injury. An individual with predominantly motor abnormalities overshadowing conceptual and symbolic disorders, is labeled "cerebral palsied." A child with little motor involvement but with a primary failure in communicative integration is called "aphasic." Where both motor and oral communicative functions are greatly disturbed, one calls the condition "cerebral palsy plus aphasia." Specific involvement of the language centers in the brain as indicative of childhood aphasia can certainly explain many of the abnormalities in language maturation.

Lastly, mental retardation frequently found in the child with cerebral palsy can certainly prevent progress in language development. Karlin and Strazzulla (15) show a direct relationship between intelligence quotients and the development of words and language.

The intelligibility of the individual is partly measured by whether his oral communication is understandable to others. One of the problems with the cerebral-palsied child is that his speech is frequently not understood. Wolfe's (16) study shows that in his experience forty-five per cent of those children with cerebral palsy have speech which is either partly understood or not understood at all. The athetoids exhibit the greatest difficulty in communicating. Other investigators agree with Wolfe's findings.

SPECIFIC SPEECH DISORDERS

Articulatory Defects

Dysarthria is one of the more common specific speech disorders found in cerebral palsy. It is due to a neuromuscular involvement of the organs of articulation. Dysarthria can be found in any of the types of cerebral palsy: the athetoid, the spastic, those children with tremors, and those demonstrating marked flaccidity.

Wolfe (16) shows that from thirty-one to fifty-nine per cent of the children studied by him have dysarthria. Dysarthria is most commonly found in the athetoid group. In the athetoid, the muscles of respiration, voice production, and articulation may be involved. Speech may, therefore, be arhythmic or jerky. Clicks and noises resulting from uncontrolled movements may be present.

The spastic cerebral-palsied child shows slow and labored speech. In the spastic, smooth motor function is difficult to achieve due to the frequent hypertonic state of the musculature and the lack of proper reciprocal innervation.

The ataxic child has difficulty in proper positioning and directional orientation. Thus, there is incorrect approximation of the structures of the speech mechanism for proper enunciation. Dysarthric speech, therefore, develops.

The defects in articulation in cerebral palsy may be either functional or organic in origin. With some children, the disorder may be so pronounced that speech is practically unintelligible. Investigators have studied the articulation of the various types of cerebral palsy. Van Riper states that both spastics and athetoids have difficulty with sounds requiring fine coordination, and find tongue-tip sounds especially difficult. Rutherford (17) states that the athetoid usually can perform movements of the tongue, lips, and jaw for speech, but that few of these movements will be under constant control. Contrary to the athetoid, however, the spastic may be limited in the direction and extent of movement of the speech organs, but his control is not impaired. The ataxic, with his defective feedback mechanisms, has little awareness as to whether he has made the appropriate response.

It is also interesting that the articulation of sounds is not consistent and that the production of a sound may be more or less intelligible depending upon where it occurs in the word, phrase, or sentence. Investigators show that the production of a sound in the initial position is easier than the production of the same sound in the medial and final positions.

Mecham, Berko, and Berko (10) state that there is almost universal agreement on the following characteristics of articulation in the child with cerebral palsy. First, tongue-tip sounds and those requiring fine coordination are the most difficult. Second, more omissions occur than substitutions or distortions. Third, action of the tongue is usually the most difficult of all speech movements. Fourth, the final sound position is more difficult than the initial or medial ones. Lastly, articulation is inefficient. A sound may be produced in the easiest possible manner, and if it serves its purpose, its use is continued even though it might not be the best that the child can do.

Since proper articulation is a problem with the cerebral-palsied child, he tends to use words of one syllable or words with stress on the initial syllable. This characteristic reduces the intelligibility of speech.

Respiratory and Voice Disorders

Normally, respiration for the production of language is modified in order for oral communication to be understandable. The respiratory cycle is, therefore, altered to consist of quick inhalations followed by more prolonged expirations.

In cerebral palsy, the child frequently retains the very rapid and irregular rhythm of respiration found in the infant. This type of breathing can last for many years after a normal child has learned to acquire a more efficient, physiologic type of respiration. The infantile breathing found in cerebral palsy leads to reduced pulmonary capacity and wasted, uncoordinated muscular activity. Both conditions result in more effortful and less efficient speech.

Palmer (18) states that over seventy per cent of the breathing anomalies in CP are found in athetoid children. In athetosis, the regulation of the respiratory system by the central nervous system is affected as a result of damage to the basal ganglia and to the hypothalamus. Koven and Lamm (19) believe this is usually a consequence of cerebral anoxia at birth.

Children with cerebral palsy have difficulty in phonation. There is great variability in their ability to voice and prolong sounds. Their problems may be in any or all of the attributes of voice: namely; pitch, intensity, quality, and variation. In the athetoid, the voice is weak and may have irregular spurts of intense volume coupled with involuntary diaphragmatic spasms. The final sounds of words and final words of phrases are often whispered. Monotones are common in the speech of the athetoid.

If spastic paralysis affects the laryngeal muscles, the vocal cords will be in various states of abnormal tension. The result is that the cords are slow in movement when sounds are to be voiced. The muscles that tighten and loosen the vocal cords may be hypertonic, resulting in difficulty when the level of pitch requires change. In cases of flaccidity, phonation may be difficult under stress situations.

A common voice problem in cerebral palsy is that of hoarseness, especially pronounced in the male child. This condition usually results from tension in the vocal cords.

In general, the incidence of both respiratory and voice disorders is much higher in the athetoid group than in any of the other types of cerebral palsy. The rate of speech production is also much slower in this group as a whole.

Stuttering

There seems to be a higher incidence of stuttering in cerebral palsy than in the normal population. Similarities exist between the general rhythm disorders found in cerebral palsy and those found in stuttering. The differential diagnosis of stuttering blocks, and spasms resulting from neuromuscular involvement of the muscles of articulation in CP, is often difficult. Rutherford (17) finds twice as many stutterers among children with cerebral palsy as among the defective speech classes in the Minneapolis public school system. Van Riper believes that under periods of emotional stress, the child with cerebral palsy often produces articulatory contacts so hard that stuttering ensues.

THERAPY

The treatment of the multiple speech disorders in cerebral palsy can be divided into three parts. First, the question of *preventive therapy*. Second, one must discuss general measures to enable the child to increase both *psychological* and *physiological readiness* for speech. Third, specific *speech measures* must be considered that are designed to improve upon the individual speech problems enumerated previously.

Preventive Therapy

One must begin to treat cerebral palsy very early if one is to obtain desirable results. The task of preventive therapy is largely the province of the parents. Perkins and Garwood (20) state that parents should be made aware of the importance to speech development of exercising their child's oral musculature by encouraging vigorous chewing, sucking, and swallowing. Second, they should stimulate the child's curiosity and help him to establish healthy social relations with children outside the home. If parents foster a sense of independence, more can frequently be accomplished in the early years to correct speech than can be expected of the best clinical regimen during the remainder of the child's life.

The results of overly protective care can militate against the future rehabilitation of speech. Obviously, the speech musculature will have little opportunity to develop. A child who is too sheltered rarely has a chance to play and, therefore, the arms and legs suffer disuse atrophy. Overprotection frequently means that psychic development may never progress beyond the early symbiotic relation with the mother.

Keeping the child in a perpetual state of infantilism is one of the serious drawbacks to the growth and development of a child with cerebral palsy. Many parents, even those of normal children, hesitate about letting their children grow up. The tendency to keep the multi-handicapped, cerebral-palsied child in an infantile stage is indeed great, since his ability to keep up with normal children is seriously compromised. If the child with CP has everything done for him, there will be little stimulation for the development of oral communication. Speech is a means by which the youngster develops independence. It is also true that with independence, the child may be stimulated to express himself more adequately.

Psychological and Physiological Readiness

It is insufficient to teach the child adequate sound production. The clinician must also attempt to increase the psychological need for speech and language. Increasing the need for speech involves teaching emotional stability and broadening the social environment as well as providing for successful experiences in speech.

A relaxed atmosphere is essential for the treatment of speech defects in the cerebral-palsied child. Evans (21) believes that there are three methods to be followed in the treatment of speech defects in cerebral palsy. First, relaxation; second, *relaxation;* and third, RELAXATION. This statement is particularly true for the athetoid, although it may represent a slight exaggeration for the other types of cerebral palsy.

Normal functioning of the chewing, sucking, and swallowing mechanisms is an aid to the development of good speech. As was said in an earlier chapter, the organs used for the production of oral communication have been "borrowed" from their more basic and primitive use of respiration and deglutition. Palmer (22) reiterates the importance of the chewing, sucking, and swallowing functions in the development of speech in cerebral palsy. A number of methods have been used in which feeding has been modified by putting the child in various postural positions.

Drooling can be one of the most difficult physiological problems preventing adequate speech development. Since children with cerebral palsy have frequent sensory involvement, many of them are not conscious of the fact that they are drooling. If the child can be taught to swallow often and to be conscious of saliva running over the lips, he frequently can learn to control the amount of drooling. Learning to keep saliva in the rear of the mouth where it can be more easily swallowed is of benefit.

SPECIFIC SPEECH THERAPY

Speech therapy can be conducted on an individual basis or as part of group therapy. The question is often raised as to which is the better method to employ. By and large, if the child with cerebral palsy exhibits severe motor impairment, a plan involving individual therapy is best. If the handicaps are less pronounced, it may be possible to work the cerebral-palsied child into a group with other speech defective children. Such placement is desirable for a child whose prospects for a normal school setting are good.

The criteria for placing cerebral-palsied children in group therapy are not always easy to formulate. Mecham, Berko, and Berko (10) believe that I.Q. and motor involvement have been overused as criteria for placing children together. They believe a good index of social competence can be obtained through the use of the Vineland Social Maturity Scale. The neurologist, orthopedist, psychologist, speech clinician, and physical therapists as well as the parents, should all be familiar with each other's appraisal of the child's capabilities. Thus, a complete profile is obtained as a guide to what attributes the child possesses for the acquisition of speech.

Respiratory Improvement

Correct breathing is important for the development of good speaking habits. Adequate breathing for speech in the child with cerebral palsy has as its goal a smooth and even exhalation of air for at least ten seconds.

The child with the athetoid type of cerebral palsy has perhaps the greatest difficulty with breathing. As a result of loss of neuromuscular coordination, the breathing of the athetoid is frequently irregular, jerky, and often asynchronous. One method of developing steady prolongation of the exhaled breath is to have the child try to keep the flame of a candle bent slightly without blowing it out. A more advanced method is to have the subject attempt to keep a piece of paper against the wall by blowing on it.

Not only is it important to develop an even, smooth exhalation of air, but one must also acquire an improved rate and rhythm of breathing if one is to speak well. A useful method in cerebral palsy is exercising voluntary breathing to the accompaniment of a ticking metronome.

Berry and Eisenson (13) stress the importance of coordinating respiration with phonation and articulation in speech. Thus, training in the *p* sound can be performed by having the child "puff" out the flame of a candle. The *b* sound can be added by having the child turn on the "motor" (voice) as he does the *p* sound. Other plosive sounds can be taught by a modification of the same procedure with the use of different parts of the articulatory system. Fricatives and sibilants are taught by restricting the exhaled breath stream in various ways.

Voice Therapy

The components of the voice include pitch, intensity, quality, and variation. In most speech defects, it is possible to analyze each of the components and determine whether deficiencies exist. It is also possible to train the individual parts of the voice so as to use stress and intonation to make speech more meaningful. Similarly, in the cerebral palsied, one can work with the individual components of voice, provided the neuromuscular dysfunction is not too great. With those children having very severe motor impairments, the segmentation of, and the training in, the various voice components become difficult.

Westlake (23) states that the cerebral palsied as a group tend to be "silent." This tendency makes it difficult for these children to initiate sounds. Westlake suggests playing the game of *secrets* as a technique to initiate voiced sounds and to encourage more vocal play.

Many investigators stress the importance of babbling and vocal play in normal growth and development of speech and language. The cerebral-palsied child who is delayed in his speech development should be encouraged to babble and to vocalize. Cuddling, caressing, and greater attention paid to the child by the parents frequently lead to greater vocalization. The imitation of animal sounds such as "moo," "bow-bow," and "baa" which are composed of the bi-labial sounds and vowels, is good for the very young child because these sounds are easy to produce. Unless the cerebral-palsied child has marked neuromuscular dysfunction preventing voice production, he will respond vocally to these animal imitations since they are concrete and interesting.

The athetoid may experience periods of abnormal laryngeal tension, especially under great emotional stress. The voice may be jerky, may crack, or may even fail completely in the middle of a word or sentence. As a result, speech is frequently produced as a series of isolated words or incomplete word groups. In such instances, therapy should be channeled into methods providing for greater relaxation and less emotional strain.

The spastic type of cerebral-palsied child usually presents difficulty in variation of voice quality. If hearing is not impaired, greater variation can be taught. Training consists of alternating the voice, first very soft and then very loud in order to hear and feel differences in intensity.

Choral speaking and group singing are important adjuncts in voice therapy. They produce good rhythm and are also combined activities which can further aid in social intercourse. These methods tend to reduce the conspicuousness of each member of the group. It is frequently the best method to use for the shy child who will not participate in conversational speech.

Methods to Improve Articulation

The articulatory organs must function properly in order that good articulation may take place. A prerequisite for adequate articulation is the ability to open and close the jaw. Secondly, the child must gain good tongue control in order to gain proficiency in the intricate characteristics of sound production. The fact that the cerebral-palsied child has articulatory defects is proof that he already possesses a functional vocabulary upon which to work.

Many cerebral-palsied children hold the mouth in an open position. The cause is either functional or organic in origin. Westlake (23) describes the *extensor thrust* in which excess neuromuscular activity makes it difficult to close the mouth voluntarily. This condition is of frequent occurrence in the athetoid. It typically involves excessive lowering of the mandible and protrusion of the tongue. Exercises are available in which the child is taught to move the mandible as well as to close the mouth. Furthermore, elevation of the tip of the tongue is one of the most difficult articulatory problems for the cerebral palsied. Here too, exercises are available to make tongue-tip skills easier to perform.

In the correction of articulatory defects, one is often asked about which sounds to work with first. In general, a good rule to follow is to teach first those sounds which are easiest to produce. The *p, b,* and *m* sounds are perhaps the easiest sounds for most children to make. The most difficult sounds to produce should be taught last, namely, those sounds requiring tongue-tip and fine, coordinated movements.

Various methods are used to establish correct sound formation. Three of these techniques will be discussed: the *stimulus-response* method, the *phonetic-placement* method, and the *moto-kinesthetic* method.

The method of stimulus-response incorporates visual, auditory, and kinesthetic avenues for stimulation. The therapist and child seat themselves in front of a mirror. The therapist repeatedly stimulates the child with the sound to be considered. The child is encouraged to listen to the sound and to watch the therapist's face as the sound is produced. The sound is then repeated by the child.

The phonetic-placement method goes one step further. In addition to incorporating the techniques used in the stimulus-response method, it adds verbal instructions by the clinician concerning where to place the articulatory organs of speech. For example, the following is often said, "Close the lips tightly and then make them explode."

Young (24) is responsible for the development of the moto-kinesthetic method. It may be used by itself or with either one of the previously mentioned techniques. The method is very effective if both touch and kinesthetic senses are intact. It often holds the attention of brain-damaged children better than other modalities of sensory stimulation. The method employs manipulation of the articulatory musculature through the actual movements of speech production.

The development of the moto-kinesthetic method revolutionized thinking about motor-speech training for the cerebral palsied. Much of the earlier muscle training in cerebral palsy was directed toward the neuromuscular system as an isolated entity, a one-way system proceeding from the stimulus to the response. The use of the moto-kinesthetic system implies that the motor disabilities of cerebral palsy are a part of the larger sensory-motor disturbances. The current view is that the central nervous system can no longer be considered a one-way process, receiving stimulation from the senses and discharging into the muscles.

Rather, many of its activities can best be explained on the basis of a circular process in which impulses emerge from the nervous system into the muscles and then re-enter the nervous system through the sense organs and proprioceptors.

Finally, once proper articulation of a sound is achieved, that sound must become a routine part of daily speech activity. When the child is able to produce the given sound in isolation successfully and easily, it must then be incorporated into the broader speech patterns of words and sentences. In order to apply the skills learned, the *speech arts* consisting of choral speaking, creative dramatics, and group discussion for the older child may be used both for enjoyment and speech improvement. Only when the sound becomes part of effective oral communication can one say that the goal of proper articulatory therapy has been achieved.

THERAPY IN HEARING

Mention must be made of the general measures incorporated in auditory training for those children with cerebral palsy who exhibit hearing problems.

Hearing disability is quite common in cerebral palsy. Hearing loss may range from a mild deficit of fifteen to twenty-five decibels to a severe loss of sixty decibels. Generally speaking, a child with a loss of over sixty decibels warrants the same consideration afforded a child with very severe hearing loss.

Mecham, Berko, and Berko (10) discuss three therapeutic measures for cerebral-palsied children exhibiting hearing problems: first, training in speech development; second, auditory training; third, speech reading.

Methods of speech development have already been discussed. The moto-kinesthetic method has been found useful for many hard-of-hearing children whose kinesthetic senses are intact. Before initiating a course in speech training, however, the child should be exposed to an abundance of auditory and visual stimulation. Auditory stimulation frequently is given with the aid of amplification.

The goal of auditory training is to allow the child to make the best possible use of his residual hearing. This objective may be realized both through methods of amplification and through training the child to listen and to discriminate more selectively and accurately. Hearing aids are commonly used as the means of amplifying sound.

If the listening intelligibility of the child is greatly reduced, speech reading should accompany speech therapy and auditory training.

SUMMARY

Speech and language problems in children with cerebral palsy are numerous and complex. The development of speech in the cerebral palsied is frequently delayed from two to four years. Furthermore, the speech which does develop is usually difficult to comprehend. The underlying organic neuromuscular brain damage occurring in cerebral palsy added to the tremendous psychological problems which arise, provide the setting for multiple speech disorders. Chief among these problems can be listed reduced articulatory ability and intelligibility, voice and breathing irregularities, disorders of rhythm and rate, symbolic functions, and problems in hearing acuity.

REFERENCES

(1) Little, W. J.: On the Influence of Abnormal Parturition, Difficult Labors, Immature Birth, and Asphyxia Neonatorum, on the Mental and Physical Condition of the Child, Especially in Relation to Deformities. *Tr. Obst. Soc. London,* 3:293, 1862.

(2) Phelps, W. M.: *Let's Talk About Cerebral Palsy.* New York, United Cerebral Palsy Associations, Inc., 1946.

(3) Phelps, W. M., and Turner, A.: *The Farthest Corner.* Chicago, National Society for Crippled Children and Adults, Inc., 1945.

(4) Cardwell, V. E.: *Cerebral Palsy—Advances in Understanding and Care.* New York, Association for the Aid of Crippled Children, 1956.

(5) Hopkins, T. W., Bice, H. V., and Colton, K. G.: *Evaluation and Education of the Cerebral Palsied Child.* Washington, D. C., International Council for Exceptional Child., 1954.

(6) Rutherford, B. R.: Extraneous Movements in Cerebral Palsy. *Physiotherapy Rev.,* 25:63, 1945.

(7) Hardy, W. G.: Testing the Hearing of Cerebral Palsied Children. *Proc. Scientific Sessions Am. Acad. for Cerebral Palsy*, 17, 1950.

(8) Saltzman, M.: *Clinical Audiology.* New York, Grune & Stratton, 1948.

(9) Goodhill, V.: Nuclear Deafness and the Nerve Deaf Child: the Importance of the Rh Factor. *Tr. Am. Acad. Ophth. & Otolar.* 54:671, 1950.

(10) Mecham, M. J., Berko, M. J., and Berko, F. G.: *Speech Therapy in Cerebral Palsy.* Springfield, Thomas, 1960.

(11) Wepman, J. M.: Speech Therapy for Cerebral Palsy Patients. *Physiotherapy Rev., 21:*82, 1941.

(12) West, R., Ansberry, M., and Carr, A.: *The Rehabilitation of Speech.* New York, Harper & Bros., 1957.

(13) Berry, M. F., and Eisenson, J.: *Speech Disorders.* New York, Appleton-Century-Crofts, Inc., 1956.

(14) Rutherford, B. R.: *Give Them a Chance to Talk.* Minneapolis, Burgess Publishing Co., 1956.

(15) Karlin, I. W., and Strazzulla, M.: Speech and Language Problems of Mentally Deficient Children. *J. Speech & Hearing Disorders,* 17:286, September, 1952.

(16) Wolfe, W. G.: A Comprehensive Evaluation of Fifty Cases of Cerebral Palsy. *J. Speech & Hearing Disorders, 15:*234, 1950.

(17) Rutherford, B. R.: A Comparative Study of Loudness, Pitch, Rate, Rhythm, and Quality of the Speech of Children Handicapped by Cerebral Palsy. *J. Speech Disorders, 9:*263, 1944.

(18) Palmer, M. F.: Speech Therapy in Cerebral Palsy. *Pediatrics, 40:*514, 1952.

(19) Koven, L. J., and Lamm, S. S.: The Athetoid Syndrome in Cerebral Palsy: Part II. Clinical Aspects. *Pediatrics, 14:*181, 1954.

(20) Perkins, W. H., and Garwood, V. P.: An Approach to Speech Therapy for the Cerebral-Palsied Individual. In, Travis, L. E.: *Handbook of Speech Pathology.* New York, Appleton-Century-Crofts, Inc., 1957.

(21) Evans, M. F.: Problems in Cerebral Palsy. *J. Speech Disorders, 12:*87, 1947.

(22) Palmer, M. F.: Speech Disorders in Cerebral Palsy. In, *Proceedings Cerebral Palsy Institute, 47.* Edited by M. Abbott. New York, Assoc. for the Aid of Crippled Children, 1950.

(23) Westlake, H.: *A System for Developing Speech with Cerebral Palsied Children*. Chicago, National Society for Crippled Children and Adults, Inc., 1951.

(24) Young, E. H., and Hawk, S. S.: *Moto-kinesthetic Speech Training*. Stanford, Stanford University Press, 1955.

Chapter 15

SPEECH DISORDERS IN
EMOTIONAL DISTURBANCES

CHILDHOOD is a collective term. It includes all ages between
the neonatal period and the termination of puberty. It carries
the individual from a condition of complete biological helplessness to the threshhold of self-dependence and creative activity.

Socialization is the outstanding achievement at the end of
this span. One may distinguish three characteristic periods of
childhood: first, the period of elementary socialization; second,
the period of domestic socialization; third, the period of com-
munal socialization. Speech and language form the means by
which the child acquires socialization. The adjustment of the
child to people and to objects in his immediate environment is
accomplished through the mediation of language, both oral and
written. A lack of socialization and communication forms one of
the hallmarks of the emotionally disturbed child.

It is fortunate that full-fledged childhood psychoses are not
very common in infancy and early childhood. As a matter of fact,
at one time, they were believed to be non-existent. The psychoses
in children as well as other forms of emotional disturbances in
the young, can be classified as language disorders. Some children
do not use their auditory mechanism because they are emotionally
disturbed. They may exhibit, therefore, what is called psychic
deafness. The childhood emotional disturbances to be discussed
are *infantile autism, childhood schizophrenia, obsessional and
anxiety neuroses.*

INFANTILE AUTISM

The diagnosis of autism has now become so popular that it is
sometimes made too quickly and hence, often erroneously. The
condition is actually rather rare. This disturbance is considered
a form of psychosis in the very young. It was first described by
Kanner (1) in 1943.

277

Infantile autism begins in very early life. Unlike the childhood schizophrenic, such a child does not participate in a period of normal emotional growth and development and then regress. The autistic child's disorders are pronounced from the preverbal age and thereafter. Because the child's history does not show periods of relative normalcy, some physicians conclude that the condition is one derived from cerebral malformation. However, no organic deprivation has been found in the autistic child. Furthermore, autistic children exhibit behavior that is significantly different from brain-damaged children.

Symptoms and Signs

Autism is characterized by two salient components without whose presence the diagnosis should not be made. First, there is extreme solitude. The withdrawal tendencies of autistic children can be noted as early as in the first year of life. The common denominator in all these cases is an inability to relate, in the ordinary way, to people. The autistic child can relate, however, to objects. This serves as one of the differentials between autism and schizophrenia. Second, there is a desire for the preservation of sameness. The child's behavior is governed by an anxious, obsessive desire to prevent change. Departures in routine can drive him to despair. The tendency toward sameness forces the child to cling to a mechanical routine and a compulsively repetitious mode of life.

Autistic children develop a good relationship with objects while being complete strangers in the world of people. They may handle toys with considerable skill. However, they see the world as a series of fragments rather than as a coherent whole. The autistic child pays no attention to persons or to the activity of people around him. Conversation in his presence holds no interest for him. Kanner (1) states that parents of autistic children refer to them as always having been "self-sufficient," "like in a shell," "happiest when left alone," "acting as though people weren't present" and "giving the impression of silent wisdom."

The parents of an autistic child frequently present him to the pediatrician as a case of hearing disability. The question of auditory loss occurs because the child fails to respond adequately to parental command. Because of low quotients in psychometric tests, some diagnosticians have also erroneously classified autistic children as examples of mental retardation. Cases are on record in which autistic children have been considered to have peripheral deafness and, therefore been assigned to schools for the deaf. The confusion of infantile autism with peripheral deafness is not infrequent since the child is often mute. Furthermore, the question of aphasia must also enter into the differential diagnosis.

An interesting observation is that many of these children are offspring of highly intelligent parents. Kanner (2) observes that the parents frequently are from professional groups consisting of teachers, physicians, and artists. Kanner also finds a high incidence of aloofness between parents and offspring. Mahler (3) points out, however, that not all parents of autistic children lack affection for their child.

Some autistic children acquire the ability to speak, while others remain mute. Language, even when present for a period of years, does not serve to convey meaning to others. *Naming* of objects may present no difficulty. Even long and unusual words may be retained with remarkable facility. Some have excellent rote memory for poems and songs. Even the mute autistic child may surprise observers by occasionally uttering single words. Kanner (1) observes that when sentences are formed, they are, for a long time, parrot-like repetitions of word combinations. They are sometimes echoed immediately, but they are just as often "stored away" by the child and voiced at a later date. One may, if one wishes, speak of *delayed echolalia.*

Affirmation is indicated by the literal repetition of a question. "Yes" is a concept that takes these children many years to acquire. One child learned to say "yes" when his father told him that he would put him on his shoulders if he said "yes." This word then came to mean only the desire to be put on his father's shoulders. It took many months before the child could detach the word "yes" from this specific situation. It took much longer before he was able to use the word as a general term of assent. To the autistic child, a meaning of a word becomes inflexible and cannot be used with any but originally acquired connotations.

The absence of spontaneous sentence formation and the echolalic type of reproduction give rise to a peculiar grammatical phenomenon. Personal pronouns are repeated just as heard. The mother says to the child, "I will give you your milk." The child expresses his desire for the milk by repeating the same words and he comes to speak of himself as "you" and of the person addressed as "I." Not only the wording, but even the mother's intonation is retained. If the mother's original remark was made in the form of a question, it is reproduced with the inflection of a question.

CHILDHOOD SCHIZOPHRENIA

Bender (4) defines childhood schizophrenia as, "a form of encephalopathy appearing at different points in the developmental curve, interfering with the normal developmental pattern of the biological unit and the social personality in a characteristic way and, because of frustration, causing anxiety to which the individual must react according to his own capacities." The psychotic involvement in schizophrenia appears somewhat later than in the autistic child who shows his deviations at a very early age.

Symptoms and Signs

The mental illness of schizophrenia occurs primarily in youth and early adult life. Bender (4), Despert (5), Lourie (6), and Pearson (7) all give adequate descriptions of the etiology and nature of the schizoid personality. Pearson (8) observes that all psychotic behavior at the childhood level is usually termed schizophrenia. He makes the further observation that schizophrenic children have had an intense fear of sounds during infancy.

The youngsters, mostly older children, usually make reasonably good adjustment prior to their illness. At first, they do not give the impression of being abnormal. They get along well at home and at school. At one point, however, they develop a marked drop in scholastic efficiency. These children begin to exhibit acute anxiety, disturbances in speech, occasional hallucinations, and loss of contact with people and with the environment. The symptoms and signs of schizophrenia finally become evident. They include seclusiveness, irritability, daydreaming with physical inactivity, bizarre behavior, and consistent lack of emotional rapport.

Two types of schizophrenic behavior are most common in children. First, there is the *hebephrenic* reaction. The child begins to lie in bed throughout the morning, lacks interest in his appearance, and becomes dull and lethargic in his actions. The youngster appears silly, giggles, and frequently carries on a hallucinatory conversation with apparent pleasure or amusement. Second, there is *simple dementia praecox*. Here, the symptoms and signs are less marked but similar to that of the hebephrenic personality. To this is added thoughts usually centering around sexual behavior. For both types, there may be a two-year prodromal period of mild depression. The catatonic and paranoid types of schizophrenia are not generally found in children.

Because the schizophrenic child lacks the appropriate response to auditory stimuli, he is often considered to have peripheral deafness. Therefore, in all cases of apparent hearing disability in the child, the pediatrician should be aware of the possibility of psychic deafness in which the auditory problem is on the basis of an emotional disorder.

As was mentioned previously, Pearson states that marked fear of sound develops early in life. During infancy, reality might have been too demanding and as a result there develops a lack of response to sound. A typical history of schizophrenia is that the child at first uses hearing and develops some use of verbal language. At about the age of eighteen to twenty-four months, however, the child gradually becomes withdrawn with a decrease in the use of speech and hearing. It is during this period, when he lacks continued development in speech, that the parents frequently believe their child is developing peripheral deafness.

A withdrawal from reality forms one of the fundamental characteristics of the schizophrenic personality. The child is bizarrely out of contact with his environment. It is at this time that the adolescent begins to experience auditory hallucinations. Oddly enough, after speech and hearing are given up in the external environment, they are frequently reinstated subjectively through hallucinations for purposes of fantasy and unrealistic behavior.

The discrepancy between mood and thought is often very striking. Fantasies or tortures may be felt or reported without the slightest outward sign of happiness or suffering. The fantasies may take the form of delusions.

Verbal expression may appear incoherent and irrelevant. Speech becomes unintelligible because of chopping up of existing words, the condensation of several words or the creation of new words *(neologism)*. The disconnection of speech may go so far as to consist of apparently unrelated words often repeated a number of times *(verbigeration, word salad)*. Speech may be extremely sparse or extraordinarily rapid. There may be *echolalia* at an age when this is no longer normal, such as after three years.

The schizophrenic personality may have two types of onset. There may be an acute beginning or a slower, more insidious appearance of the disturbance. Furthermore, the older the child at the onset of the illness, the more closely do the clinical features resemble the adult pattern.

MISCELLANEOUS EMOTIONAL DISTURBANCES RELATED TO SPEECH

Early infantile autism and childhood schizophrenia are the most common types of psychoses in childhood producing impairment in speech and language development. In addition, there are other emotional disturbances encountered in children which influence speech development. These are called the neuroses and consist mainly of *anxiety* and *obsessional states*.

Relinquishing the use of speech and hearing is an effective way for the child to prevent anxiety-producing stimuli from overwhelming him. Anxiety states usually do not cause the severe incapacities found in children with psychoses such as childhood schizophrenia and early infantile autism. Furthermore, the speech and hearing disabilities are often situational and intermittent.

Situational conditions which produce inhibition of speech and hearing are not common in the child below the ages of four or five years. Their most frequent occurrence is above the age of six. Apparently, the very young child does not differentiate between situations as far as speech and language are concerned.

Obsessional neurosis is characterized by rigid adherence to a certain orderly routine. Frequently, obsessions in childhood are related to an inordinate desire for cleanliness. There may be lack of normal speech and language formation. However, the lack of verbal communication associated with cases of obsessional neurosis is not as complete as that found in autism or schizophrenia. In general, the neuroses are much less disabling for the organism than are the psychoses.

DIFFERENTIAL DIAGNOSIS

Two types of differential diagnoses must be made. First, differences must be pointed out among the various types of emotional disturbances themselves. Second, a differential must be found between the emotional disorders and the organic disabilities. Those organic conditions to be considered in a differential diagnosis include childhood aphasia, mental retardation, and peripheral deafness (see discussion of differential diagnosis in the chapter on aphasia). Because the psychoses and neuroses are basically disorders of personality, the best differential diagnosis is made on the basis of varying behavioral patterns.

All the psychological disorders occurring in childhood and influencing speech development have a fundamental common denominator. The child behaves primarily on the basis of subjective stimulation in which the environment no longer is involved as a determinant of behavior. This lack of environmental influence is basic to the emotionally disturbed child. Children with aphasia, mental retardation, and peripheral deafness do not relinquish contact with the environment. As Myklebust (9) points out, the behavior of a child with organic deficiencies is characterized by the way in which he *attempts to relate* to his environment. The behavioral symptomatology of the emotionally disturbed child is characterized by the manner in which he *dissociates* himself from the environment and behaves as if the only stimulation of consequence is that which comes from within. He essentially denies the external world.

SPEECH AND LANGUAGE DEVELOPMENT

There is no orderly development of speech in the emotionally disturbed child. Frequently there is complete lack of verbal communication as is characteristic of infantile autism. As Kanner points out, however, some autistic children speak quite freely. Contrary to the autistic child, the schizophrenic shows normal development of speech and language during the first year of life. It is at the age of one to two years that speech development ceases in childhood schizophrenia. While mutism is common in cases of psychic deafness, it is quite rare in aphasia, mental retardation, and peripheral deafness. Marked mutism is, therefore, a cardinal sign of emotional involvement in childhood. The child with psychic deafness is, perhaps, the most speechless of children having auditory disorders.

The reason for lack of speech in the autistic and schizophrenic child is that the environment no longer influences the child's behavior. Therefore, verbal communication as the means of relating the environment to the individual is no longer necessary.

Some schizophrenic children vocalize in a bizarre manner, somewhat analogous to aphasic behavior. Bender (10) states that if one wishes an opportunity to observe the greatest number of aphasic anomalies in early childhood, one can find them in the schizophrenic child. She observes that it almost seems that the schizophrenic child plays with the various types of aphasic disorders. At times, children with schizophrenia can speak normally and then become aphasic, going through the various types of aphasic behavior.

In an attempt to remain an integral part of the environment, the aphasic may use jargon speech and the child with peripheral deafness may use his voice projectively. However, the emotionally disturbed child usually does neither. Autistic children relate well to objects, such as blocks, but they do not vocalize while engaging in activity with such objects. The schizophrenic child is more vocal, but his vocalizations usually derive from internal fantasy and relate to neither objects nor people. Furthermore, when autistic or schizophrenic children do use words, they are not for purposes of communication.

The responses of children with psychic deafness are character-istic in that these children seem to hear but do not respond to auditory stimuli. Unlike the aphasic child who gives inconsistent responses to auditory stimuli, the emotionally disturbed child will usually reject the auditory world. Schizophrenic children, espe-cially, respond poorly to auditory stimulation. Sullivan (11) de-scribes this quality of schizophrenic behavior. Loud intensities do not change the child's responsiveness. Characteristically, autistic and schizophrenic children lack response to auditory stimuli regardless of the level of intensity.

Myklebust (9) feels that many emotionally disturbed children with psychic deafness do not use speech echolalically, since these children are often mute. He further notes, however, that some autistic children do engage in an echolalic type of speech. Clini-cally, it appears that autistic children who engage in echolalia have not completely rejected people and the environment as much as those who do not. By reacting echolalically, the child can maintain a minimum of contact with people and with the auditory world. Myklebust (9) states that from the point of view of auditory disorders, echolalia signifies integrity of the auditory mechanism. He feels it should be considered symptomatic of conditions other than peripheral deafness.

McGinnis (12) states that if one is to find any semblance of schizophrenia in aphasic children, one would be more likely to find it in the echolalic type of sensory aphasic without motor involvement.

Lack of Non-verbal Communication

The ability or inability to use gestures as a means of language communication is important as a differential diagnostic feature between nonorganic and organic disorders. In emotionally dis-turbed children, there is a lack in the use of gestures as a form of communication. The autistic child does not point to a person. His rejection of reality is characteristically in the area of human relations. He maintains contact with objects in his environment and treats people as though they are also inanimate. Since human beings are regarded as lifeless, the autistic child has no use for the development of gestures or speech as a means of communication.

The schizophrenic child, like the autistic child, does not use gestures. Myklebust (9) states that the schizophrenic has not only rejected the people of his world, but he has rejected the inanimate objects as well. He says that while the schizophrenic child might engage in manipulation of an object, the object is not used meaningfully. Such complete withdrawal obviously makes gestures and language impossible for communication purposes. Myklebust continues by saying that such children might use speech and language internally. This is revealed by changes in facial expression.

Eisenson (13) observes that very often schizophrenic children use human beings as things rather than as people. They relate to people as if they were inanimate, and often, in spite of the way they relate, one cannot tell what kind of object the person is supposed to represent.

Facial Expression

Aphasic children attempt to use visual clues, including facial expression, as a mode of action even though they are largely unsuccessful. Children with peripheral deafness are able to use such clues as a source of contact with the environment. Emotionally disturbed children, however, characteristically ignore face to face contact. The autistic child exhibits this sign to its fullest extent. His rejection of people is signified by the rejection of people's faces. Schizophrenic children also have characteristics in which they reject people's faces. While the autistic child refuses to look at the face, the schizophrenic will look at the face without recognition or awareness. It is as though he looks through the face. Children with anxiety states or less extensive emotional disorders do not reject facial contact in the above manner. Although they do manifest fear of face to face contact, they will relate more satisfactorily and they will make use of facial expression as a guide to action.

Autistic children usually do not smile, laugh or cry. Schizophrenic children do smile and laugh, but only in a bizarre manner. They engage in smiling and laughter for fantasy only. They laugh and cry only in a preoccupied, detached manner and only as a result of subjective stimulation.

Laughing and smiling are responses of normal human beings to reactions of people around them. Such behavior reflects psychological integrity and well-being. Crying is a normal reaction in children when they feel threatened or are in pain. The significance of crying is that many autistic and some schizophrenic children do not cry even when injured. This reduction of sensitivity to pain is direct evidence of their lack of response to environmental stimuli, even at painful thresholds.

Lack of Use of Compensatory Mechanisms

Furthermore, children with emotional disorders do not use visual or tactile clues as compensatory mechanisms. Ordinarily, children with speech and hearing impairment on an organic basis, will develop their sense of sight and their sense of touch to a very keen level, in an effort to compensate for their deficiency. Indeed, although aphasic children cannot compensate effectively for their lack of adequate speech, they do not reject environmental sensory stimulation. Therefore, when a child exhibits a speech or hearing problem and other sensory avenues are not used to compensate for it, the presence of a psychological disorder should be considered. When a two to three-year-old child demonstrates a complete lack of adequate response to variable types of sensory stimuli in the external environment, and when no plausible organic cause can be given, the presence of childhood schizophrenia must be seriously entertained.

Motor and Play Activities

The depression of motor activity in the schizophrenic child is very well presented by Bender (4). The motor behavior of both schizophrenic and autistic children includes ritualistic and stereotyped activities. They might rock themselves while in a standing position, remain in a fixed position for an unusual period of time, or twirl themselves incessantly, without regard to their surroundings. According to Bender (10), the lack of patterned behavior is the most characteristic part of schizophrenia. This is present to some degree in every area of activity. This is the key to the diagnosis of schizophrenia.

Play activities give one a chance to observe the child's ability to socialize. Aphasic children make the attempt to play, but they cannot grasp the total situation. Children with peripheral deafness engage in social play when their activities are essentially visual. Autistic children engage in play, but it is not social play. Kanner (14) states that they are greatly attracted to blocks. Kanner points out that they form intricate designs and patterns with these blocks, possessing an unusual memory for what they have constructed. The building with blocks is stereotyped, perseverative, and repetitious.

Schizophrenic children do not engage in play activities. They may go through the motions of playing, but they will not relate emotionally to the activity.

The child with an anxiety disorder usually exhibits social awareness and does participate in play activities. However, in severe anxiety states these children may also retreat into themselves and reject the external environment.

TREATMENT

The treatment for the severe emotional disorders of early infantile autism and childhood schizophrenia is for the most part psychiatric. Since these disorders are frequently progressive mental aberrations, they can be carried over into adult life. Early treatment is, therefore, imperative. It remains for child psychiatry and clinical psychology to emphasize the development of nonverbal psychotherapeutic techniques.

Few authorities use shock therapy as part of the treatment for childhood schizophrenia. Most feel that this treatment should not be used with children. Even if shock therapy is instituted, its effect is not nearly as rewarding a therapeutic agent in the child as it is in the adult.

A recent and very successful approach in the treatment of emotional disorders in childhood is *educational therapy*. In both public and private schools, small special classes have been organized for these children. Appropriate methods and materials have been devised to help the disturbed child become oriented to his environment. The goal of educational therapy is to bring order into the disordered mind of the child through an organized program of suitable instruction and play.

This chapter has dealt with functional emotional disturbances in childhood. It is necessary to point out, however, that organic disorders such as aphasia, cerebral palsy, deafness, and cleft palate, in addition to causing communication difficulties, result in emotional disturbances in children. The organic component of these disorders can frequently be treated, thereby decreasing the emotional stress. Furthermore, such disorders as stuttering and voice problems, which have both organic and non-organic components, may cause emotional problems or may be the result of emotional difficulty. Thus, both aspects of these disorders must be treated.

REFERENCES

(1) Kanner, L.: Autistic Disturbances of Affective Content. *Nervous Child*, 2:217, 1943.

(2) Kanner, L.: *Child Psychiatry*. Springfield, Thomas, 1948.

(3) Mahler, M. S.: On Child Psychosis in Schizophrenia; Autistic and Symbiotic Infantile Psychosis. In, *Psychoanalytic Study of the Child*, 7:286. New York, International Universities Press, 1952.

(4) Bender, L.: Childhood Schizophrenia. *Am. J. Orthopsychiat.*, 17:40, 1947.

(5) Despert, L.: Psychotherapy in Childhood Schizophrenia. *Am. J. Psychiat.*, 104:36, 1947.

(6) Lourie, R. S., Pacella, B. L., and Piotrowski, Z. A.: Studies on the Prognosis in Schizophrenic-like Psychoses in Children. *Am. J. Psychiat.*, 22:542, 1943.

(7) Pearson, G. H. J.: *Emotional Disorders of Children*. New York, W. W. Norton, 1949.

(8) Pearson, G. H. J.: A Survey of Learning Difficulties in Children. In, *Psychoanalytic Study of the Child*, 7:366. New York, International Universities Press, 1952.

(9) Myklebust, H.: *Auditory Disorders in Children*. New York, Grune & Stratton, 1954.

(10) Bender, L.: *Panel Discussion on Childhood Aphasia.* Palo Alto, Stanford University Institute on Childhood Aphasia, September, 1960.

(11) Sullivan, H.: *The Interpersonal Theory of Psychiatry.* New York, W. W. Norton, 1953.

(12) McGinnis, M.: *Panel Discussion on Childhood Aphasia.* Palo Alto, Stanford University Institute on Childhood Aphasia, September, 1960.

(13) Eisenson, J.: *Panel Discussion on Childhood Aphasia.* Palo Alto, Stanford University Institute on Childhood Aphasia, September, 1960.

(14) Kanner, L.: Early Infantile Autism. *J. Pediatrics,* 25:211, 1944.

Chapter 16

RELATED LANGUAGE DISABILITIES

LANGUAGE SKILLS

THERE are four basic language skills: *listening, speaking, reading,* and *writing.* Listening and speaking are acquired before the child attends school. Reading and writing are usually learned at school.

Listening as a language skill means the active focusing of attention on spoken language and the comprehension of the speech uttered. Comprehension calls forth response, either mental, verbal, or physical. Speaking is the utterance of verbal symbols arranged in an appropriate order to convey thought processes. Listening and comprehension of oral language precede speaking.

Reading and writing skills are usually acquired at the same time while the child is receiving formalized school training. Reading consists of both the focusing of attention through the visual sense on symbols located on a written page, together with the comprehension of these symbols. Writing is the reproduction of visual symbols placed in an appropriate order to express thoughts. Listening and silent reading are both sensory processes involving *comprehension* of language. Speaking and writing are both motor processes involving *production* of language. Furthermore, listening and speaking are concerned with sounds, while reading and writing are concerned with letters that represent sounds.

PERCEPTION AND PRODUCTION OF LANGUAGE

The eye and the ear compose the peripheral sensory organs concerned with the perception of both written and oral language. It is through the eye and the ear that the infant first receives sensory impulses such as visual and sound stimulation. Orton (1) separates perception of language following peripheral reception into three stages or levels. First, is the *arrival platform,* which is the primary cortical sensory area. Second, is the undifferentiated *gnostic area.* The third and highest level is the differentiated area which is concerned with *symbolization* and its expression.

According to Orton, sensory impulses received by the eye and ear terminate in that area of the cortex which has been called the arrival platform. At the second, higher level, these impulses are formulated into concepts. Here, the impulses become patterned into knowing or gnostic forms capable of recall by the psychic process called memory. At the highest level, there is further refinement into concept formulation and symbolization which is so necessary for the productive language faculty.

The preceding paragraphs discuss the increasing complexity of sensory development. In the motor sphere, there is a similar arrangement in order of increasing integrative complexity. At the lowest level, motor pathways are formed once the infant learns to contract striated muscle voluntarily. At the second level, the child acquires the ability to perform planned, purposeful movements. Finally, at the highest level, the youngster learns to express himself through meaningful speech and language. (See chapter 9, Fig. 33, page 145.)

Disturbances in the natural order of sensory and motor language integration lead to many disabilities. Loss of primary perception (cortical blindness or deafness) results from a lesion at the first sensory level. Visual and auditory agnosia develop from involvement at the second level. Receptive aphasia, or loss of concept formation, takes place from a disturbance at the highest sensory level. Lesions at the first level on the motor side result in anarthria. Apraxia develops at the second level of motor involvement. Finally, expressive aphasia results from involvement at the highest motor level. (See chapter 9, Fig. 34, page 147.)

The separation of the sensory functions of language perception into three stages or levels is the result primarily of clinical observation. However, investigators have accumulated much anatomical data which substantiate the existence of these levels. *Microscopic* studies of these areas present differences in size and in the arrangement of the nerve cells. Furthermore, differences in the order and time of *myelinization* of many cerebral areas provide evidence for the existence of the three levels. Since myelinization is directly related to the establishment of function, its time of appearance in differing anatomical sites in the central nervous system can serve as a useful means in judging the maturation of cerebral areas. Flechsig found that myelinization proceeds in three distinct waves. He demonstrated that at birth, only the arrival platform or first cortical level receives myelin. A second period of myelinization follows during the first three months of life, at which time deposition of myelin takes place around the arrival platforms. It is only during the final or third wave that maturation occurs in the areas of the third level.

ACQUIRING LANGUAGE SKILLS

In the normal course of language development, the average child listens and slowly comprehends the language used around him. Thus, he acquires a stock of sounds which will later be used to form words that have meaning. Soon, in imitation of people in his environment, he produces these sounds as words. Later, he learns to place the words together in an appropriate order and to change forms of words to express more fully his desires and feelings.

Glanzer (2) cites two aspects in the child's development of language. These consist of: a) the rules, structures, and transformations that make up the *syntax of the language;* b) the classes of items, or *parts of speech,* that the syntax orders. Glanzer quotes Braine's (3) work involving the extensive recording of word combinations uttered by children over a period of several months. Recordings were started from the time the child possessed an estimated vocabulary of ten to twenty single-word utterances and before the appearance of the first word-combination.

Braine (3) studied a twenty-three-month-old child who used the verbs *do, get, want, find,* and *eat* with nouns. The words *there, here,* and *that* were also used with nouns. Thus, both verbs and adverbs are used with nouns at this age. At twenty-five months, the same child put questions and statements in the same word order, but he differentiated questions from statements by using a rising intonation for the former. For example, the child might say, "Me go?" with an up glide, asking the question of whether he is going to be taken out. Similarly, he may say, "Me go" with a down glide, indicating his intention to go out with the family. As the child grows older, "grammatical categories are increasingly better defined and more extensive, and dominate speech performance."

By the time the child is ready for school, he has learned to speak in phrases and sentences. He may also have learned some letters of the alphabet and to read a few words. Some children learn to print letters and to print their names before entering school.

It is the task of the school to teach the child reading and writing and to develop further the skills of listening and speaking. Since language is the instrument of learning, through the teacher's speech and through books, development of language skills is basic to the education of the child.

RELATED LANGUAGE DISABILITIES

Related language disabilities will be discussed in the order in which the child first acquires the language skills. Thus, difficulties arising from faulty aspects of listening, speaking, reading, and writing will be treated in this order.

Listening Disabilities

Various auditory handicaps were listed in the chapters concerning aphasia and hearing disorders. Peripheral hearing loss causes the child to be deprived of the sensory intake of sound. Central deafness occurs when the child can hear, but because of cortical lesions, he cannot comprehend what is heard. The term dysacusis is used to describe a defect in audition which is usually central and on an integrative or interpretive level.

Wernicke's auditory area in the superior temporal gyrus of the cerebral cortex is designated as area 41. It is surrounded by the psychoauditory zone, area 42. (See chapter 5, Fig. 17.) The auditory word area concerned with memories of words heard is located in the second temporal gyrus. It is the critical area for understanding words and sentences. The destruction of this area will cause auditory aphasia. Mental retardation will also cause impaired comprehension of spoken language.

Speaking Disabilities

Speaking, the second language skill, may be delayed for many reasons as has been discussed in earlier chapters. Some of the causes consist of auditory disorders, mental retardation, impairment of the central nervous system such as cerebral palsy, lesions in the motor speech areas, and emotional or functional disturbances.

The motor speech area is called Broca's area. It is located at the posterior end of the inferior frontal convolution and is designated as area 44. Its destruction causes motor aphasia or loss of the ability to speak. In many cases, the parents are the first to become concerned when the child fails to speak at the normal age. Delay in speech development requires special treatment by qualified speech pathologists and clinicians.

Since listening and speaking comprise the subject matter of this book and have been discussed in previous chapters, the related language skills of reading and writing together with their disabilities will be more fully discussed below.

Reading Disabilities

There are many causes for a delay in learning to read. Marked deficiencies in visual acuity may underlie such a difficulty. If errors in refraction, congenital cataracts, corneal opacities, or central chorioretinitis are the causes, they should be thoroughly investigated and corrected, if possible. Defects of hearing also lead to poor auditory discrimination of words. In some cases, poor reading appears to have its roots in residuals of an uncorrected word deafness. A general intellectual defect is also a frequent cause of failure in reading. Emotional disturbances, as exhibited in antagonism toward teachers, apathy toward school work, or lack of adequate disciplinary training at home, may all play their part. Finally, as Orton (1) states, "When all of such factors are excluded, there remains a group of very considerable size in every school who have shown no evidence of any delay or abnormality in either their physical, mental, or emotional development until they have reached school and are confronted with reading, and then they suddenly meet a task which they cannot accomplish."

Reading has been described as the process of decoding visual symbols that represent sounds in words. The visual word area is concerned with storing memories of words seen. It is located in the angular gyrus, Brodman's area 39, and its immediate surroundings. Destruction of this area will cause *alexia* or *word blindness*. Its integrity is essential to skill in reading.

Reading difficulties have been the concern of educators all over the world. In recent years, especially in the United States and England, there has been some criticism of the teaching of the related language skills of reading and writing to children in the primary grades.

In cases where myelinization has been thought to be delayed, investigators have found some children unable to recall the details of symbols and their sequences. Thus, *w, m, u,* and *n* are confused because of their form similarities. There is also right-to-left confusion in which *b* and *d,* and *p* and *g* are misread. The disability in sequence of symbols consists in a sinistral progression instead of the usual dextral. This may affect the reading of a whole word or part of a word.

Monosyllabic words may be fairly well handled in some types of reading disabilities, whereas words of two or three syllables may be badly confused. Such difficulties may not be constant or fixed. In children with this disability, mirror writing with its sinistral progression may be much better performed than the usual dextral writing.

Pathology in Reading Disabilities

Orton (1) believes that congenital disorders causing defects in symbolization are due to variations and delays in the acquisition of dominance by one cerebral hemisphere. These delays in language development are abetted by mistraining and occasionally by disease or injury to the brain. The loss of symbolic formation and expression is a form of aphasia.

It is stated by Orton (1) that the capacity to comprehend the meaning or purpose of objects seen is usually retained in patients who have lost the capacity to read. Thus, Orton presents three brain levels at which sensory stimuli may be incorrectly tabulated. At the lowest level, one finds *cortical blindness,* in which there is no conscious vision. At the second level, one speaks of *mind blindness,* in which the child sees so that he does not collide with objects in the environment, but is quite unable to recall the purpose or use of the objects seen. At the highest level, one has *word blindness (alexia),* in which there is no loss of vision or of the capacity to recognize and interpret objects, but in which reading, as exhibited by the printed word, does not convey its meaning. The latter condition will cause serious reading disability.

Orton (1) states that in order to produce cortical blindness, the appropriate cortical area in *both* cerebral hemispheres has to be destroyed at the primary arrival platform. Similarly, in order to produce mind blindness, the majority of investigators believe that bilateral destruction is necessary at the second or undifferentiated gnostic level. Word blindness is caused by a lesion in the highest differentiated area concerned with symbol formation. It is sufficient in this case to have lesions in only one hemisphere, provided it is the dominant hemisphere. Injury here will cause disorders of both spoken and written language.

Many investigators believe word blindness to be associated with a lack of lateral dominance. In many children with reading disabilities, there is no clear-cut preference for the right or left hand. Frequently, even when the child seems to exhibit a definite preference as to eye or foot laterality, no conclusion can be drawn concerning his handedness. In spite of the fact that there seems to be a clinical association of reading disorders with lack of cerebral dominance, some authorities believe that laterality is not a significant factor in reading dysfunction.

Measuring Reading Ability

Since the ability to read depends upon the ability to see, a great deal of attention has been given to the reader's eyes.

Normally, in reading, there is a *fixation area* in which the eye absorbs the word or words. The eye then shifts slightly to the right until the next series of words appears to be focused on the macula area of the retina. When the end of a line is reached, the eyes sweep diagonally from right to left to take up fixation at the beginning of the next line. This is known as the *return sweep*. The *recognition span* is the average number of words seen and assimilated in one fixation. At times, the eyes may move too far to the right when attempting to view the next set of words. This necessitates a slight shift back to the left in order to view a part of the line that has been missed. This action is called regression. The area that is seen to the right and left of the point of fixation is called the *visual span*.

As the child matures in his ability to read, he spends less time on fixation, makes fewer regressions and performs eye movements in a more efficient and decisive manner. Individuals vary in both the visual span and the recognition span.

Special eye tests have been devised to determine various functions of the eyes. Naturally, adequate binocular visual acuity is a prerequisite for good reading. The *telebinocular* visual survey uses a special type of stereoscope through which cards are viewed to measure acuity of vision, coordination, fusion, depth perception, and color blindness. The *ophthalmograph* is employed to record eye movements on a graph while the child reads. A beam of light is directed into the eyes and is reflected from the cornea. This is photographed on a moving film by a camera.

Teaching Reading

It is the opinion of many reading experts that a great majority of children who have reading problems are not organically or intellectually impaired. Many defects in reading have been attributed to conflicting theories in regard to teaching reading.

When the average child arrives at school, he can comprehend and produce spoken language. How is reading related to the sounds he knows and uses in words? Written English is highly unphonetic. Yet the alphabet presumably represents sounds. How can the child decode these letters or printed symbols into sounds that represent words as he knows them?

There are two basic methods of teaching reading to the child in the United States; the earlier *phonic method* and the later *word recognition method*.

Phonic Method. The phonic method was the first system used in teaching reading. The phonic method breaks a word up into its component sounds and syllables. It has continued in use in many areas of the country.

The phonic method is based upon the child's learning the alphabet and reading the words aloud so that he can associate sound with meaning. When the youngster begins to attend school, he brings with him the language skills of listening and speaking. He has already associated sound with meaning. In the phonic method, this association is continued by breaking down the printed word into familiar sounds. Thus, an easy transition is provided between the listening and speaking language skills learned at home, and the reading and writing skills acquired in school.

Word Recognition Method. During the third decade of the twentieth century, some educators decided that the process of learning to read could be simplified and speeded up if the word recognition method of teaching were used.

The entire word is seen and recognized, without its being broken down into its component parts. In this method, visual association with meaning takes precedence over association of sound with meaning. The difficulty here is that the child cannot make use of the language skills of listening and speaking that he has already acquired at the preschool level.

The word recognition method gained popularity in what was called at the time, progressive education. This method emphasizes silent reading for comprehension, rather than oral reading for both sound and comprehension. It consists of recognizing the word visually by its configuration and not by breaking down the word into its component sounds and syllables. As a result of teaching recognition of whole words, difficulties in spelling arise.

The word recognition method was taught widely for some time until many parents and educators became alarmed at the number of children who could not learn to read. At present, many educators are returning to the phonic method of teaching reading. A lively controversy has been waged for some time over both these methods of teaching reading. In many areas, experiments are being made using a combination of the phonic and word recognition methods.

The present trend in the teaching of reading is to use phonics or sound as a method. A national survey conducted by Harvard University on a Carnegie Foundation grant showed that no school system today completely omitted phonics as an aid to teaching reading.

Initial Teaching Alphabet. Since there are only twenty-six letters in the alphabet and forty sounds in the language, it is impossible to write words the way they sound. In England, the new ITA (Initial Teaching Alphabet) has been used to overcome the confusion caused by the unphonetic spelling found in the English language. According to reports, the experiment has met with success in expediting reading.

The Initial Teaching Alphabet is composed of forty-four letters that represent the vowels, diphthongs, and consonants of the language. Children begin to learn reading skills using primers printed in this new forty-four-letter, phonetic alphabet. It has been emphasized that this is an alphabet just for beginning readers and is to be used only for the purpose of teaching reading. Once this has been accomplished, the ITA is discarded. This alphabet is now being used as an experimental method in various areas of the United States.

A recent survey of the National Council of Teachers of English, involving approximately 4,000,000 pupils, showed an overwhelming number of children to be poor readers according to standardized tests. The results indicated that thirty-five per cent were seriously retarded. Of these, only sixteen per cent were retarded because of mental deficiency and other forms of brain damage. Reading is therefore still a major concern in most school systems.

Bilingualism

Bilingualism is a frequent cause of reading disability in a second language. In many large cities of the world, children attend schools where subjects are taught in a language other than their mother tongue. When Puerto Rican children, for example, settle in continental United States, they are taught subjects in English, although in Puerto Rican schools they are taught in Spanish. English is taught as a second language on the island.

The change in the language of instruction naturally causes retardation in the language skills in English. Listening (comprehension), speaking, reading, and writing are all below grade level. Children all over the world who are in schools that use a language other than their mother tongue have the same initial handicap.

Relationship Between Speech and Reading

There have been many studies concerning the relationship be-between speech proficiency and abilities in other language skills. Carroll (4) quotes Williams and Schneiderman as finding "substantial relationship between articulatory ability and other indices of language ability."

Tureen (5) studied the relationship between speech and reading ability, as well as the effects of speech therapy on reading. In two groups each of forty speech defective children from grades two to six, Tureen found a positive relationship between speech defects and reading disability. The more severe the speech defect, the greater the reading difficulty. The study also showed that in the experimental group, speech therapy facilitated improved reading as well as decreased the speech defect.

Writing Disabilities

The motor area for writing is located at the posterior portion of the second frontal convolution, just anterior to the motor area of the arm. A lesion in this area will cause motor agraphia, or loss of the ability to write.

Adequate functioning of the central nervous system depends upon the interaction of both the sensory and motor systems. The complex process of writing also depends upon intact sensory and motor functions. The three sensory levels of perception for the comprehension of the written word have already been discussed. The lowest level receives the sensory impression. The second, higher area involves the recognition of what is seen. The most advanced level is concerned with concept formulation and symbolization. Writing involves the integrity of all these steps in comprehending language, plus the production of language made visible through the use of the motor area for writing.

There are various degrees of rapidity with which children learn to read and write. Often this has little relationship to the general intelligence of the child. Some children use mirror writing. This form of disability evidences itself in movement from right to left instead of from left to right. These children print the word *cat* as *taɔ*.

Agraphia, the inability to write, is infrequently seen alone since its anatomical representation encompasses a very small area near the centers that control movement of the hands and the centers for speech production. Agraphia may coexist with reading disability and its associated difficulty in spelling. Problems in reading and writing are, therefore, very closely allied. Usually, children are taught reading and writing at the same time.

Orton (1) devotes a great deal of consideration to handedness and the shifting of handedness in children with writing problems. In many cases of agraphia, there is a history of a shift from the left to the right hand in early infancy, or an enforced training of the right hand for writing in spite of a strong preference for the left. The left-handed child is at a disadvantage in learning to write. Orton states, however, that "a proper position of the paper and hand will greatly facilitate the acquisition of left-hand writing both in the case of left-handed children who are just learning to write and in the mistrained left-handers who are experimenting with a shift. The proper position of the paper is the exact mirror opposite of that employed for right-handed children, that is, with the top of the sheet inclined toward the right."

SOCIAL, EDUCATIONAL, VOCATIONAL, AND EMOTIONAL PROBLEMS RELATED TO LANGUAGE DISABILITIES

Since language is the tool of communication, instruction, and learning, any disability in this area will cause severe social, educational, vocational, and emotional problems.

A diagnosis of the cause of the language disability is necessary for the most successful treatment of the difficulty. It must be remembered, however, that in many cases of reading deficiency and articulatory disorders, there appears to be no readily identifiable cause. It is important in such cases to begin remedial measures even though the exact etiologic mechanism of the difficulty is not known. Postponement of remedial work may cause delay in the acquisition of related language skills and, therefore, delay in educational progress. Difficulty in these areas will cause social maladjustment for the pupil in school and in his community. The emotional problems that result will make remedial measures more complex. Authorities agree that efforts to remedy the deficiencies should begin as early as possible.

REFERENCES

(1) Orton, S. T.: *Reading, Writing, and Speech Problems in Children.* New York, W. W. Norton, 1937.

(2) Glanzer, M.: Toward a Psychology of Language Structure. *Speech Hearing Res.,* 5 No. 4:303, December, 1962.

(3) Braine, M. D. S.: On Learning the Grammatical Order of Words. *Psychol. Rev.,* in press.

(4) Carroll, J. B.: Language Development. *Encyclopedia of Educational Research,* p. 744. New York, The Macmillan Co., 1960

(5) Tureen, J.: *An Investigation of the Relationship Between Defects of Speech and Reading Achievement, Including a Study of the Effects of Speech Therapy on Reading Achievement.* Unpublished Ph.D. thesis, New York University, 1958.

INDEX

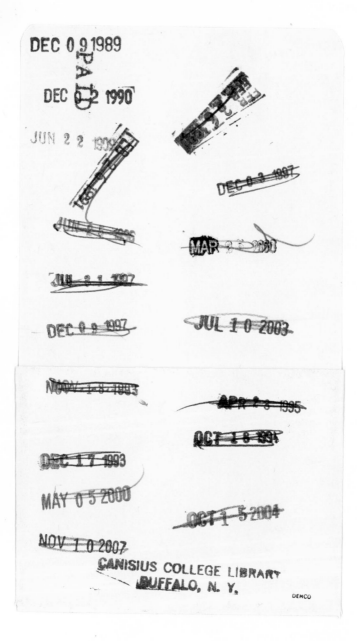